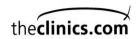

theclinics.com

CLINICS IN CHEST MEDICINE

Controversies in
Mechanical Ventilation
GUEST EDITOR
Neil R. MacIntyre, MD

June 2008 • Volume 29 • Number 2

SAUNDERS

An Imprint of Elsevier, Inc.
PHILADELPHIA   LONDON   TORONTO   MONTREAL   SYDNEY   TOKYO

W.B. SAUNDERS COMPANY

A Division of Elsevier Inc.

Elsevier Inc. • 1600 John F. Kennedy Boulevard • Suite 1800 • Philadelphia, Pennsylvania 19103-2899

http://www.chestmed.theclinics.com

CLINICS IN CHEST MEDICINE
June 2008
Editor: Sarah E. Barth

Volume 29, Number 2
ISSN 0272-5231
ISBN-13: 978-1-4160-5867-0
ISBN-10: 1-4160-5867-2

Reprints: For copies of 100 or more, of articles in this publication, please contact the Commercial Reprints Department, Elsevier Inc., 360 Park Avenue South, New York, New York 10010-1710. Tel. (212) 633-3813; Fax: (212) 462-1935; e-mail: reprints@elsevier.com.

The ideas and opinions expressed in *Clinics in Chest Medicine* do not necessarily reflect those of the Publisher. The Publisher does not assume any responsibility for any injury and/or damage to persons or property arising out of or related to any use of the material contained in this periodical. The reader is advised to check the appropriate medial literature and the product information currently provided by the manufacturer of each drug to be administered to verify the dosage, the method and duration of administration, or contraindications. It is the responsibility of the treating physician or other health care professional, relying on independent experience and knowledge of the patient, to determine drug dosages and the best treatment for the patient. Mention of any product in this issue should not be construed as endorsement by the contributors, editors, or the Publisher of the product or manufacturers' claims.

Clinics in Chest Medicine (ISSN 0272-5231) is published quarterly by Elsevier Inc., 360 Park Avenue South, New York, NY 10010-1710. Months of issue are March, June, September, and December. Business and Editorial Offices: 1600 John F. Kennedy Blvd., Suite 1800, Philadelphia, PA 19103-2899. Customer Service Office: 6277 Sea Harbor Drive, Orlando, FL 32887-4800. Periodicals postage paid at New York, NY and additional mailing offices. Subscription prices are $232.00 per year (US individuals), $370.00 per year (US institutions), $113.00 per year (US students), $255.00 per year (Canadian individuals), $444.00 per year (Canadian institutions), $149.00 per year (Canadian students), $297.00 per year (international individuals) $444.00 per year (international institutions), and $149.00 per year (international students). International air speed delivery is included in all *Clinics* subscription prices. All prices are subject to change without notice. **POSTMASTER:** Send address changes to *Clinics in Chest Medicine*, Elsevier Periodicals Customer Service, 6277 Sea Harbor Drive, Orlando, FL 32887-4800. Customer Service: 1-800-654-2452 (US). From outside the United States, call 1-407-563-6020. Fax: 1-407-363-9661. E-mail: JournalsCustomerService-usa@elsevier.com.

Clinics in Chest Medicine is covered in *Index Medicus, Current Contents/Clinical Medicine, EMBASE/Excerpta Medica, Science Citation Index,* and *ISI/BIOMED.*

Printed in the United States of America.

GUEST EDITOR

NEIL R. MACINTYRE, MD, Professor of Medicine, Division of Pulmonary and Critical Care Medicine, Duke University Medical Center, Durham, North Carolina

CONTRIBUTORS

JENNIFER BECK, PhD, Department of Newborn and Developmental Paediatrics, Neonatal Intensive Care Unit, Sunnybrook Health Sciences Centre; Department of Pediatrics, University of Toronto, Toronto, Ontario, Canada

RICHARD D. BRANSON, MSc, RRT, Associate Professor of Surgery, University of Cincinnati, Cincinnati, Ohio

JESSICA Y. CHIA, MD, Department of Medicine, Division of Pulmonary and Critical Care Medicine, Duke University Medical Center, Durham, North Carolina

ALISON S. CLAY, MD, Assistant Professor, Departments of Surgery and Medicine, Duke University Medical Center, Durham, North Carolina

KENNETH DAVIS, Jr, MD, Professor of Surgery and Anesthesia, University of Cincinnati, Cincinnati, Ohio

RAJIV DHAND, MD, Professor of Medicine, and Division Chief, Division of Pulmonary, Critical Care, and Environmental Medicine, University of Missouri; Staff Physician, Harry S. Truman Veterans' Affairs Hospital; Medical Director of Respiratory Care, University of Missouri Hospitals and Clinics, Columbia, Missouri

E. WESLEY ELY, MD, MPH, Associate Director for Research, VA Tennessee Valley Geriatric Research, Education and Clinical Center (GRECC), VA Service, Department of Veterans Affairs Medical Center; Professor of Medicine, Division of Allergy, Pulmonary, and Critical Care Medicine, Center for Health Services Research, Vanderbilt University School of Medicine, Nashville, Tennessee

TIMOTHY D. GIRARD, MD, MSCI, Instructor in Medicine, Division of Allergy, Pulmonary, and Critical Care Medicine, Center for Health Services Research, Vanderbilt University School of Medicine, Nashville, Tennessee

JOSEPH GOVERT, MD, Associate Professor of Medicine, Division of Pulmonary, Allergy and Critical Care Medicine, Duke University Medical Center, Durham, North Carolina

VAMSI P. GUNTUR, MD, Assistant Professor of Medicine, Division of Pulmonary, Critical Care, and Environmental Medicine, University of Missouri; University of Missouri Hospitals and Clinics, Columbia, Missouri

DEAN R. HESS, PhD, RRT, Assistant Director of Respiratory Care, Respiratory Care, Massachusetts General Hospital; Associate Professor of Anesthesia, Harvard Medical School, Boston, Massachusetts

CHRISTOPHER KING, MD, Fellow, Pulmonary/Critical Care Medicine, Walter Reed Army Medical Center, Washington, District of Columbia

NEIL R. MACINTYRE, MD, Professor of Medicine, Division of Pulmonary and Critical Care Medicine, Duke University Medical Center, Durham, North Carolina

LISA K. MOORES, MD, Assistant Dean for Clinical Sciences, and Professor of Medicine, The Uniformed Services University of the Health Sciences, Bethesda, Maryland

ROBERT L. OWENS, MD, Clinical and Research Fellow, Department of Medicine, Pulmonary and Critical Care Unit, Massachusetts General Hospital; Instructor, Harvard Medical School, Boston, Massachusetts

GHEE-CHEE PHUA, MBBS, MRCP, FCCP, Associate Consultant, Department of Respiratory and Critical Care Medicine, Singapore General Hospital, Singapore

CHUIN SIAU, MBBS, MRCP, Interdepartmental Division of Critical Care Medicine, University of Toronto, Toronto, Ontario, Canada

CHRISTER SINDERBY, PhD, Department of Critical Care Medicine, Keenan Research Centre, Li Ka Shing Knowledge Institute, St. Michael's Hospital; Department of Medicine, University of Toronto, Toronto, Ontario, Canada

THOMAS E. STEWART, MD, FRCPC, Interdepartmental Division of Critical Care Medicine, University of Toronto; Critical Care Unit, Mount Sinai Hospital; Critical Care Unit, University Health Network, Toronto, Ontario, Canada

WILLIAM S. STIGLER, MD, Resident in Internal Medicine, Massachusetts General Hospital, Wang Ambulatory Care Center; Instructor, Harvard Medical School, Boston, Massachusetts

CONTENTS

ventilated in such a way as to minimize alveolar over-distension and repeated alveolar collapse. Clinical trials have used such lung protective strategies and shown a reduction in mortality; however, there is data that these "one-size fits all" strategies do not work equally well in all patients. This article reviews other methods that may prove useful in monitoring for potential lung injury: exhaled breath condensate, pressure-volume curves, and esophageal manometry. The authors explore the concepts, benefits, difficulties, and relevant clinical trials of each.

Effects of Respiratory-Therapist Driven Protocols on House-Staff Knowledge and Education of Mechanical Ventilation

Jessica Y. Chia and Alison S. Clay

High practice variability in critical care medicine contributes to medical errors and the high cost of ICU care. Clinical guidelines and protocol-based strategies can reduce the variation and cost of ICU medicine, increase adherence to evidence-based interventions, and reduce error, thereby improving the morbidity and mortality of critically ill patients. There are various barriers to guideline adherence, and protocols often are more successful when implemented by nonphysicians. However, this has potential consequences for house-staff knowledge and education. This article discusses the implications of mechanical ventilation protocols on patient care and medical education, and this article offers suggestions for synchronizing the processes for improving patient care to improve medical education.

Mechanical Ventilation in an Airborne Epidemic

Ghee-Chee Phua and Joseph Govert

With the increasing threat of pandemic influenza and catastrophic bioterrorism, it is important for intensive care providers to be prepared to meet the challenge of large-scale airborne epidemics causing mass casualty respiratory failure. The severe acute respiratory syndrome outbreak exposed the vulnerability of health care workers and highlighted the importance of establishing stringent infection control and crisis management protocols. Patients who have acute lung injury and acute respiratory distress syndrome who require mechanical ventilation should receive a lung protective, low tidal volume strategy. Controversy remains regarding the use of high-frequency oscillatory ventilation and noninvasive positive pressure ventilation. Standard, contact, and airborne precautions should be instituted in intensive care units, with special care taken when aerosol-generating procedures are performed.

Proportional Assist Ventilation and Neurally Adjusted Ventilatory Assist—Better Approaches to Patient Ventilator Synchrony?

Christer Sinderby and Jennifer Beck

Understanding the regulation of breathing in the critical care patient is multifaceted, especially in ventilator-dependent patients who must interact with artificial respiration. Mechanical ventilation originally consisted of simple, manually-driven pump devices, but it has developed into advanced positive pressure ventilators for continuous support of patients in respiratory failure. This evolution has resulted in mechanical ventilators that deliver assist intermittently, attempting to mimic natural breathing. Recently, modes of mechanical ventilation that synchronize not only the timing, but also the level of assist to the patient's own effort, have been introduced. This article describes the concepts related to proportional assist ventilation and neurally adjusted ventilatory assist, and how they relate to conventional modes in terms of patient-ventilator synchrony.

Does Closed Loop Control of Assist Control Ventilation Reduce Ventilator-Induced Lung Injury?

Richard D. Branson and Kenneth Davis, Jr

The standard of care for mechanical ventilation of the patient who has acute lung injury remains volume control ventilation at 6 mL/kg. Despite this fact, clinicians often employ pressure control ventilation and adaptive pressure control ventilation in an attempt to improve synchrony and limit the possibility for overdistension. Adaptive pressure control uses pressure control breaths to guarantee a minimum delivered tidal volume. Other techniques (such as adaptive support ventilation) use pressure-limited breaths, switching between time and flow cycling based on patient effort. Neither of these techniques has been compared with volume control in a randomized setting. Understanding operation of these techniques is essential for determining any impact on outcome or ventilator induced lung injury.

FORTHCOMING ISSUES

RECENT ISSUES

THE CLINICS ARE NOW AVAILABLE ONLINE!

Access your subscription at:
http://www.theclinics.com

CLINICS
IN CHEST
MEDICINE

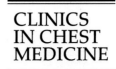

Clin Chest Med 29 (2008) xi–xii

Erratum

CT, Positron Emission Tomography, and MRI in Staging Lung Cancer

Jeremy J. Erasmus, MBBCh, Bradley S. Sabloff, MD

Division of Diagnostic Imaging, University of Texas, MD Anderson Cancer Center,
1515 Holcombe Boulevard, Unit 0371, Houston, TX 77030, USA

The above article, which appeared in the March 2008 issue ("Contemporary Chest Imaging"), contained a figure that was printed in black and white, but should have been printed in color. The figure appears in color here (see next page).

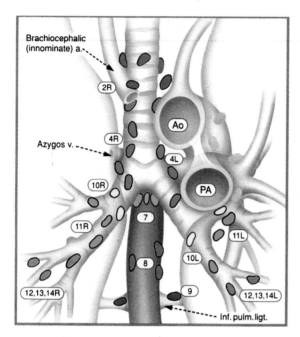

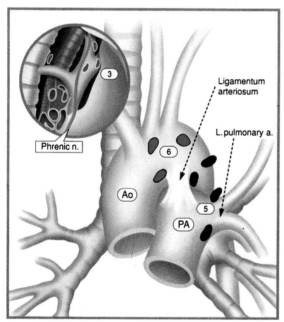

Superior Mediastinal Nodes

⬤ **1** Highest Mediastinal

⬤ **2** Upper Paratracheal

⬤ **3** Pre-vascular and Retrotracheal

⬤ **4** Lower Paratracheal
(including Azygos Nodes)

N_2 = single digit, ipsilateral
N_3 = single digit, contralateral or supraclavicular

Aortic Nodes

⬤ **5** Subaortic (A-P window)

⬤ **6** Para-aortic (ascending
aorta or phrenic)

Inferior Mediastinal Nodes

⬤ **7** Subcarinal

⬤ **8** Paraesophageal
(below carina)

⬤ **9** Pulmonary Ligament

N₁ Nodes

○ **10** Hilar

⬤ **11** Interlobar

⬤ **12** Lobar

⬤ **13** Segmental

⬤ **14** Subsegmental

ELSEVIER
SAUNDERS

Clin Chest Med 29 (2008) xiii

CLINICS
IN CHEST
MEDICINE

Preface

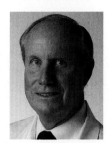

Neil R. MacIntyre, MD
Guest Editor

Mechanical ventilation has been a mainstay of respiratory life support for almost a century. For much of this time, the goal simply was to provide positive pressure breaths in sufficient numbers to maintain adequate gas exchange. Beginning in the middle of the twentieth century, additional features appeared (such as positive end expiratory pressure) to improve lung recruitment and the ability of the patient to trigger breaths to enhance comfort.

In the last two decades, however, an explosion of new concepts and new technologies has occurred. Perhaps the most important of these concepts is the notion of ventilator induced lung injury (VILI). Beginning with important animal experiments in the 1980s and 1990s and culminating in large clinical trials at the beginning of the twenty first century, the idea that inappropriate ventilator settings could kill patients went to the core of practices in widespread use at the time. No longer could the ventilator targets be simply gas exchange; the lung also had to be protected from regional overstretch and collapse/re-recruitment VILI.

At this same time, microprocessor technology opened many new capabilities to monitor respiratory function, create "customized" breath delivery patterns, and provide feedback control of many ventilator settings according to various inputs. Adjuncts for better humidification, aerosol delivery, therapeutic gas delivery, and patient positioning also appeared. Finally, novel non-convective forms of respiratory life support (such as high frequency ventilation, liquid ventilation, and easier to use extracorporeal systems) also were being developed.

Amid this bewildering array of new concepts and technologies, clinical practice is evolving and "trying to keep up." However, many questions and controversies remain on how practice should change. In this series of articles, I have asked world authorities on these subjects to address, what I consider, the most important of these controversies. These articles are designed to look at a specific controversial area and then provide a balanced assessment from the evidence available. It is hoped that the reader will see these issues more clearly, and even if answers are still not yet clear, at least have greater insight.

Neil R. MacIntyre, MD
*Division of Pulmonary and
Critical Care Medicine
Duke University Medical Center
Erwin Road
Room 1120, Box 3911
Durham, NC 27710, USA*

E-mail address: neil.macintyre@duke.edu

0272-5231/08/$ - see front matter © 2008 Elsevier Inc. All rights reserved.
doi:10.1016/j.ccm.2008.02.005

ELSEVIER
SAUNDERS

Clin Chest Med 29 (2008) 225–231

CLINICS
IN CHEST
MEDICINE

Is There a Best Way to Set Tidal Volume for Mechanical Ventilatory Support?

Neil R. MacIntyre, MD

Division of Pulmonary and Critical Care Medicine, Duke University Medical Center,
Room 1120, Box 3911, Erwin Road, Durham, NC 27710, USA

Concept of overstretch injury should guide selection of tidal volume

The lung can be injured when it is stretched excessively by positive pressure ventilation. The most widely recognized injury is alveolar rupture, presenting as extra-alveolar air in the mediastinum (pneumo-mediastinum), pericardium (pneumo-pericardium), subcutaneous tissue (subcutaneous emphysema), pleura (pneumothorax), or vasculature (air emboli) [1,2]. The risk for extra-alveolar air increases as a function of the magnitude and duration of alveolar overdistension. Thus, interactions of respiratory system mechanics and mechanical ventilation strategies (high regional tidal volume and positive end-expiratory pressure or PEEP, both applied and intrinsic) that produce regions of excessive alveolar stretch (ie, transpulmonary distending pressures in excess of 40-cm H_2O) for prolonged periods create alveolar units at risk for rupture [1,2].

In experimental animals, a parenchymal lung injury not associated with extra-alveolar air (ventilator-induced lung injury or VILI) can also be produced by mechanical ventilation strategies that stretch the lungs beyond the normal maximum (ie, transpulmonary distending pressures of 30-cm to 35-cm H_2O) [3–5]. Because the injury is a result of physical stretching, the term "volutrauma" has been coined to describe it. Pathologically, volu-trauma is manifest as diffuse alveolar damage [3–8] and seems to be potentiated by a shear stress phenomenon that occurs when injured alveoli are repetitively opened and collapsed during the ventilatory cycle [6–11].

VILI is most likely to occur clinically in lung injuries where low-resistance and high-compliance (relatively healthy) regions are interspersed with either low-compliance or high-resistance units. Under these conditions, even with a near normal sized tidal volume, the low-resistance and high-compliance units receive a disproportionately high regional tidal volume and thus are at risk for regional volutrauma (Fig. 1). This understanding is driving mechanical ventilation management strategies to reduce end-inspiratory volumes and pressures.

VILI effects are not restricted to the lungs. Numerous animal studies have confirmed that an array of inflammatory cytokines is released into the systemic circulation as a consequence of VILI [8,11–13]. Several clinical studies have indicated that this phenomenon also occurs in patients receiving mechanical ventilation at potentially injurious ventilator settings [12–14]. Another consequence of VILI seems to be the loss of the lung's bacterial barrier function. Specifically, several animal studies have shown that VILI is associated with dramatic increases in alveolar-capillary bacterial translocation [15].

These systemic effects of VILI may explain the observation that patients receiving mechanical ventilation for respiratory failure usually die from multi-organ failure and shock, not from refractory hypoxemia or acidemia. Death seems to result from the systemic effects of VILI, not from the lung disease. If VILI could be reduced, mortality might be reduced.

Comparing and contrasting trials of low tidal volume (low stretch) ventilation in acute lung injury

Observational trials from over two decades ago, using low tidal volumes and "permissive"

E-mail address: neil.macintyre@duke.edu

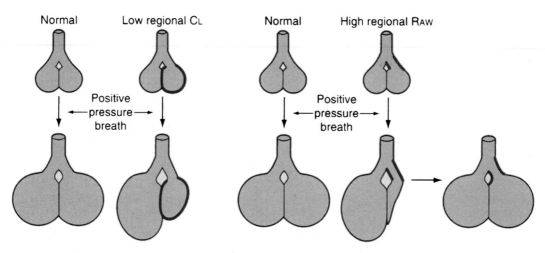

Fig. 1. Distribution of positive pressure breaths in normal lungs as compared to lungs with regional abnormalities. Note that in the presence of regional compliance (CL) or resistance (RAW) abnormalities, the breath will overinflate the healthier lung unit. (*Reprinted from* Mason RJ, Broaddus VC, Murray JF, et al, editors. Textbook of respiratory medicine. 4th edition. Philadelphia: Elsevier/Saunders; 2005; with permission.)

hypercapnia in severe acute respiratory distress syndrome (ARDS) showed benefit when compared with historical controls [16]. This led to a change in thinking about the risks of aggressively pursuing gas exchange goals if high pressures and volumes were required [17]. Since then, six randomized clinical trials have evaluated the role of tidal volume settings in the pathogenesis of VILI in patients with acute lung injury (ALI) and ARDS [18–23]. All six studies were designed to compare two differing approaches to ventilator management: a generous tidal volume approach (high tidal volume strategy) that characterized clinical practice at the time and prioritized achieving near normal alveolar ventilation and alveolar recruitment versus a restrictive tidal volume approach (low tidal volume strategy) that prioritized providing lung protection and accepted adequate, but not necessarily normal gas exchange.

In three of these trials the mortality outcome was similar in the high and low tidal volume strategies [18–20]. In the other three [21–23], a mortality benefit was associated with the use of smaller tidal volumes (Table 1). The most likely explanations for these disparate results are the tidal volume separation and the plateau pressures (a common surrogate for end-inspiratory alveolar stretching pressure) in the two tidal volume groups (see Table 1). Specifically, the tidal volume difference in the three positive trials was substantially larger than the tidal volume difference in the

three negative trials. In addition, in the positive trials, the plateau pressures in the high tidal volume group were well above 30-cm H_2O, while in the small tidal volume group these pressures were generally below this threshold. In contrast, in the three negative trials the plateau pressures were generally below 30-cm H_2O in both the high and low tidal volume groups. It should also be noted that while an aggressive PEEP strategy was also used in two of the three positive trials, the largest of the three [22] had equivalent PEEP levels in both tidal volume groups.

In many of these trials, there were trends toward more respiratory acidosis and lower levels of PO_2 in the small tidal volume groups. These effects, however, did not seem to adversely impact outcomes. In addition, there is a general sense that smaller tidal volumes might be more difficult to synchronize with patient effort. However, analysis of sedation use in the largest trial [24] showed no increase in sedative or opiate use when using the small tidal volume strategy.

Operationalizing these data

Although the general consensus now favors mechanical ventilatory strategies that prioritize limiting end-inspiratory lung stretch [17], controversy exists on how to operationalize this concept based on the results of these trials.

Table 1
Tidal volume trials in ALI and ARDS

	Tidal volume (VT) (mL/kg PBW)			Pplat (cm H_2O)		
	High VT	Low VT	Difference	High VT	Low VT	Difference
Negative studies						
Brower et al [18]	10.2	7.3	2.9	29.8	26.5	3.3
Brochard et al [19]	10.4	7.2	3.2	31.7	25.7	6.0
Stewart et al [20]	10.6	7.2	3.4	26.5	23.0	3.5
Average	10.4	7.2	3.2	29.3	25.1	4.2
Positive studies						
Amato et al [21][a]	11.9	6.1	5.8	37.0	30.0	7.0
ARDS Net [22]	11.7	6.3	5.4	32.8	24.9	7.9
Villar et al [23][a]	10.2	7.3	2.9	32.6	30.6	2.0
Average	11.2	6.6	4.7	34.1	28.5	5.6

Abbreviations: PBW, predicted body weight; Pplat, plateau pressure.
[a] Also included aggressive PEEP strategies.

Is it simply enough to limit plateau pressure?
Or does tidal volume have to be limited as well?

There is controversy about whether maximal stretch (reflected in the end-inspiratory volume and distending pressure) or the tidal stretch (reflected in the tidal volume) is the major determinant of overdistension VILI. Clearly maximal stretch is important. However, excessive tidal stretch [25,26], frequency of stretch [5,27], and rapidity of stretch (ie, high initial gas flow into the lung) [28] may also contribute to VILI.

The argument for focusing only on maximal stretch (plateau pressure) involves several points. First, there are few data from animal studies of VILI that suggest large tidal volumes in the setting of a low plateau pressure causes harm. Second, in all of the tidal volume trials described above, a consistent finding was that harm occurred only in the groups with high plateau pressures, not necessarily the groups with high tidal volumes. Third, an analysis of over a thousand eligible, but not randomized, subjects in the large ARDS Network tidal volume trial [29] suggested that tidal volumes intermediate between the two tidal volumes being studied (and perhaps adjusted to plateau pressure) had similar beneficial outcomes to the small tidal volume group. Fourth, larger tidal volumes in the setting of a plateau pressure less than 30-cm H_2O, if indeed safe, would provide more clinical flexibility in terms of patient comfort and gas exchange management.

The argument for focusing on both maximal and tidal stretch (plateau pressure and tidal volume) also involves several points. First, although nonhuman data are few, intriguing alveolar cell tissue culture stretching experiments [30] and animal hyperventilation studies [31] suggest that VILI is a result of both maximal and tidal stretch. Second, reanalysis of the largest tidal volume study to date, the ARDS Network trial [26] suggested that even in the patients with plateau pressures well below 30-cm H_2O, reductions in tidal volume seemed to provide additional benefit. Third, in several observational trials described in more detail below [32–34], the size of the tidal volume, more than the plateau pressure, was the major risk factor for the development of lung injury in patients initially receiving mechanical ventilations for reasons other that acute lung injury. Fourth, although smaller tidal volumes may limit clinical options, adequate gas exchange and reasonable ventilator synchrony was achievable in all of the small tidal volume trials.

Taken together, the available data clearly implicate maximal stretch (plateau pressure) as a major risk factor for VILI, and thus the clinical target should be below 30-cm H_2O. However, it would also seem reasonable based on the available data to recommend tidal stretch (tidal volume) reductions as well, even in the presence of a plateau pressure of less than 30-cm H_2O, unless there are compelling reasons to do otherwise.

What is a practical tidal volume approach that would use both plateau pressure and tidal volume reductions as goals?

Limiting tidal and maximal stretch must involve tradeoffs. Specifically, the need for potentially injurious pressures, volumes, and supplemental oxygen must be weighed against the benefits of gas-exchange support and muscle unloading. To this end, gas exchange goals have been reassessed over the last decade, and now pH goals as low as 7.15 to 7.20, and PO_2 goals as low as 55 mm Hg are often considered acceptable if the lung can be protected from VILI [16,17,35,36]. It is worth emphasizing that the low tidal volume strategy in the ARDS Network trial had worse gas exchange than the high tidal volume strategy, but this low tidal volume strategy had better survival [22]. Thus, the additional recruitment of injured regions from the large tidal volume strategy was likely accompanied by regional overdistension and VILI in healthier regions that led to worse survival.

Therefore, it seems reasonable to limit the tidal volume as much as possible while maintaining some minimal but adequate level of gas exchange support. An initial tidal volume of 6-mL/kg ideal body weight thus would seem to be a reasonable starting point for at least two reasons. First, this volume is close to a normal resting tidal volume in spontaneously breathing individuals. Second, it was the initial setting used in the large National Institutes of Health ARDS Network trial and was tolerated well [22].

The response to this initial tidal volume setting, however, needs to be carefully assessed. Inadequate alveolar ventilation may be addressed by rate adjustments, inadequate oxygenation may be addressed by PEEP and fraction of inspired oxygen adjustments, and discomfort may be addressed by flow manipulations or judicious sedation. If necessary, tidal volume can be increased, but this adjustment should be made cautiously, and every attempt should be made to keep end-inspiratory distending pressures as low as possible.

A plateau pressure below 30-cm H_2O is a useful target to help guide these tidal volume strategies. It is important to remember two points about this measurement. First, in the presence of stiff chest walls, the plateau pressure may be heavily influenced by chest wall mechanics and thus overestimate lung stretch (an esophageal balloon to estimate pleural pressure may be useful under these circumstances) [37]. Second, even though the normal human lung has a maximal distending pressure at total lung capacity of 30-cm to 35-cm H_2O, repetitive applications of even this normal maximal stretching pressure for prolonged periods of time may be associated with injury [31]. Also, when even the 6-mL/kg tidal volume is associated with high distending pressures, further reductions should be considered.

Is this approach for all? Or are there specific groups in whom it should be avoided?

Because low tidal volume strategies have not been prospectively studied in a randomized controlled fashion in non-ALI patients, it is difficult to give a strong evidence based recommendation. However, it is important to remember that in almost all forms of respiratory failure, lung injury is heterogeneous with very sick lung units interspersed with healthier lung units [38]. This creates a situation where positive pressure ventilation will preferentially ventilate the healthier units and potentially expose them to regional overdistention (see Fig. 1). Because the goal of low tidal volume and low plateau pressure ventilation is to protect the normal lung units from stretch injury, it would make sense to incorporate this approach in virtually all patients requiring mechanical ventilation.

There are some human trials supporting this approach. Older studies in subjects with obstructed lung disease were the first to describe the concept of "permissive" hypercapnia: strategies that reduced minute ventilation to reduce lung overdistention [39]. More recently, a large retrospective analysis of patients initially mechanically ventilated for a variety of reasons other than ALI or ARDS found that a substantial proportion of this population subsequently developed criteria for ALI while on the ventilator. In a multivariate analysis of these data, the size of the tidal volume was the strongest predictor of ALI development [33]. This same group went on to institute a small tidal volume ventilator management protocol and observed a substantial reduction in ALI developing in ventilated patients over the next several years [35]. A recent review of nine trials studying small versus large tidal volume strategies in the perioperative period showed either unchanged or reduced cytokine levels and a shorter duration of mechanical ventilation associated with the use of small tidal volumes [40]. Importantly, none of these studies suggested harm associated with small tidal volume ventilation. Clearly larger clinical trials are needed to further explore this approach [41].

One exception to small tidal volume ventilation might be in the patient with a neurologic injury. In these patients where hypercarbia needs to be avoided, higher minute ventilations (and thus tidal volumes) may be required. Another group of patients might be those recovering from respiratory failure and who have been weaned to low levels of ventilatory support (eg, 5-cm H_2O

pressure support) and who demand a tidal volume less than 6 mL/kg predicted body weight. Under these circumstances, a search should be made for treatable causes of excessive respiratory drive (eg, pain, acidosis, and other causes). However, such patients may simply be receiving unnecessary support and should be evaluated for ventilator discontinuation potential [42]. Merely sedating such patients under these circumstances to suppress respiratory drive is probably inappropriate.

What can be done when a low tidal volume and low plateau pressure strategy cannot provide adequate gas exchange?

An important clinical problem is what to do when a minimal level of gas exchange cannot be supported without violating these protective guidelines (ie, excessive plateau pressures and tidal volumes). Under these circumstances, two strategies could be considered. First, prolongation of the inspiratory time may help recruit some lung units and improve gas mixing without having to increase tidal volume or PEEP [43]. Allowing spontaneous breathing to occur during the inflation phase may further improve recruitment and reduce the need for sedation that is often required with reverse ratio (ie, inspiratory time less than expiratory time) ventilation [44,45]. Second, high-frequency ventilation can provide a high mean airway pressure to facilitate recruitment while theoretically reducing tidal and maximal stretch [46]. Both these strategies have been shown to support gas exchange well in ARDS, but no definitive outcome trials have been performed. Vasodilators could be considered under these conditions, although outcome benefits have not been studied. Finally, a recent randomized trial has demonstrated a mortality benefit to extracorporeal support in patients who have severe ARDS [47].

Summary

An inappropriate tidal volume setting can overstretch and injure the lung. Maximal stretch, tidal stretch, frequency of stretch, and rate of stretch are all implicated in such injury. Moreover, the stretch injury produces systemic injury by liberating cytokines and translocating bacteria in the lung. Clinical trials have shown that limiting maximal and tidal stretch improves outcomes, even if gas exchange is partially compromised. Current strategies should thus focus on

limiting tidal and maximal stretch as much as possible. Although changing clinical practice is often a slow process [48], there seems to be a growing awareness of overdistension injury by the critical care community and an overall trend toward reducing tidal volumes [48].

References

[1] Zwilich CW, Pierson DJ, Creagh CE, et al. Complications of assisted ventilation. A prospective study of 354 consecutive episodes. Am J Med 1974;57: 161–70.
[2] Gammon RB, Shin MS, Groves RH Jr, et al. Clinical risk factors for pulmonary barotraumas: a multivariate analysis. Am J Respir Crit Care Med 1995;152: 1235–40.
[3] Webb HH, Tierney DF. Experimental pulmonary edema due to intermittent positive pressure ventilation with high inflation pressures: protection by positive end-expiratory pressure. Am Rev Respir Dis 1974;110:556–65.
[4] Tsuno K, Prato P, Kolobow T. Acute lung injury from mechanical ventilation at moderately high airway pressure. J Appl Physiol 1990;69:956–61.
[5] Kolobow T, Morentti MP, Fumagalli R, et al. Severe impairment in lung function induced by high peak airway pressure during mechanical ventilation. Am Rev Respir Dis 1987;135:312–5.
[6] Muscedere JG, Mullen JB, Gan K, et al. Tidal ventilation at low airway pressures can augment lung injury. Am J Respir Crit Care Med 1994;149: 1327–34.
[7] Dreyfuss D, Saumon G. Ventilator-induced lung injury: lessons from experimental studies. Am J Respir Crit Care Med 1998;157:294–323.
[8] Plotz FB, Slutsky AS, van Vught AJ, et al. Ventilator-induced lung injury and multiple system organ failure: a critical review of facts and hypotheses. Intensive Care Med 2004;30:1865–72.
[9] Chu EK, Whitehead T, Slutsky AS. Effects of cyclic opening and closing at low- and high-volume ventilation on bronchoalveolar lavage cytokines. Crit Care Med 2004;32:168–74.
[10] Benito S, Lemaire F. Pulmonary pressure-volume relationship in acute respirator distress syndrome in adults: role of positive end expiratory pressure. J Crit Care 1990;5:27–34.
[11] Herrera MT, Toledo C, Valladares F, et al. Positive end-expiratory pressure modulates local and systemic inflammatory. Int Care Med 2003;29:1345–53.
[12] Trembly L, Valenza F, Ribiero SP, et al. Injurious ventilatory strategies increase cytokines and C-fos M-RNA expression in an isolated rat lung model. J Clin Invest 1997;99:944–52.
[13] Uhlig S, Ranieri M, Slutsky AS. Biotrauma hypothesis of ventilator-induced lung injury. Am J Respir Crit Care Med 2004;169:314–5.

[14] Ranieri VM, Suter PM, Totorella C, et al. Effect of mechanical ventilation on inflammatory mediators in patients with acute respiratory distress syndrome. JAMA 1999;282:54–61.

[15] Nahum A, Hoyt J, Schmitz L, et al. Effect of mechanical ventilation strategy on dissemination of intra-tracheally instilled E-coli in dogs. Crit Care Med 1997;25:1733–43.

[16] Hickling KG, Walsh J, Henderson S, et al. Low mortality rate in adult respiratory distress syndrome using low-volume. Pressure-limited ventilation with permissive hypercapnia: a prospective study. Crit Care Med 1994;22:1568–78.

[17] Slutsky AS. ACCP Consensus Conference: mechanical ventilation. Chest 1993;104:1833–59.

[18] Brower RG, Shanholtz CB, Fessler HE, et al. Prospective, randomized controlled clinical trial comparing traditional versus reduced tidal volume ventilation in acute respiratory distress syndrome patients. Crit Care Med 1999;27:1492–8.

[19] Brochard L, Roudot-Thoraval F, Roupie E, et al. Tidal volume reduction for prevention of ventilator-induced lung injury in acute respiratory distress syndrome. The Multicenter Trial Group on Tidal Volume reduction in ARDS. Am J Respir Crit Care Med 1998;158:1831–8.

[20] Stewart TE, Meade MO, Cook DJ, et al. Evaluation of a ventilation strategy to prevent barotraumas in patients at high risk for acute respiratory distress syndrome. Pressure- and Volume-Limited Ventilation Strategy Group. N Engl J Med 1998;338:355–61.

[21] Amato MB, Barbas CS, Medievos OM, et al. Effect of a protective ventilation strategy on mortality in ARDS. N Engl J Med 1998;338:347–54.

[22] NIH ARDS Network. Ventilation with lower tidal volumes as compared with traditional tidal volumes for acute lung injury and the acute respiratory distress syndrome. N Engl J Med 2000;342:1301–8.

[23] Villar J, Kacmarek RM, Pérez-Méndez L, et al. A high positive end-expiratory pressure, low tidal volume ventilatory strategy improves outcome in persistent acute respiratory distress syndrome: a randomized, controlled trial. Crit Care Med 2006;34(5):1311–8.

[24] Cheng IW, Eisner MD, Thompson BT, et al, Acute Respiratory Distress Syndrome Network. Acute effects of tidal volume strategy on hemodynamics, fluid balance, and sedation in acute lung injury. Crit Care Med 2005;33:63–70.

[25] Terragni PP, Rosbach G, Tealdi A, et al. Tidal hyperinflation during low tidal volume ventilation in ARDS. Am J Respir Crit Care Med 2007;175:160–6.

[26] Hager DN, Krishnan JA, Hayden DL, et al. ARDS Clinical Trials Network. Tidal volume reduction in patients with acute lung injury when plateau pressures are not high. Am J Respir Crit Care Med 2005;172:1241–5.

[27] Rich PB, Douillet CD, Hurd H, et al. Effect of ventilatory rate on airway cytokine levels and lung injury. J Surg Res 2003;113:139–45.

[28] Rich BR, Rickert CA, Sawada S, et al. Effect of rate and inspiratory flow on ventilator induced lung injury. J Trauma 2000;49:903–11.

[29] Eichacher PQ, Gertlenbergcr EP, Banks SM, et al. Meta analysis of ALI/ARDS trials testing low tidal volumes. Am J Respir Crit Care Med 2002;166:1510–6.

[30] Tschumperlin DJ, Oswari J, Margulies AS. Deformation-induced injury of alveolar epithelial cells. Effect of frequency, duration, and amplitude. Am J Respir Crit Care Med 2000;162:357–62.

[31] Mascheroni D, Kolobow T, Fumagalli R, et al. Acute respiratory failure following pharmacologically induced hyperventilation: an experimental animal study. Intensive Care Med 1988;15:8–15.

[32] Gajic O, Dara SI, Mendez JL, et al. Ventilator-associated lung injury in patients without acute lung injury at the onset of mechanical ventilation. Crit Care Med 2004;32:1817–24.

[33] Gajic O, Frutos-Vivar F, Esteban A, et al. Ventilator settings as a risk factor for acute respiratory distress syndrome in mechanically ventilated patients. Intensive Care Med 2005;31:922–6.

[34] Yilmaz M, Keegan MT, Iscimen R, et al. Toward the prevention of acute lung injury: protocol guided limitation of large tidal volume ventilation and inappropriate transfusion. Crit Care Med 2007;35:1660.

[35] Sinclair SE, Kregenow DA, Lamm WJ, et al. Hypercapnic acidosis is protective in an in vivo model of ventilator-induced lung injury. Am J Respir Crit Care Med 2002;166:403–8.

[36] Kregenow DA, Rubenfeld GD, Hudson LD, et al. Hypercapnic acidosis and mortality in acute lung injury. Crit Care Med 2006;34:1–7.

[37] Brander L, Ranieri VM, Slutsky AS. Esophageal and transpulmonary pressure help optimize mechanical ventilation in patients with acute lung injury. Crit Care Med 2006;34:1556–8.

[38] Nieszkowaska A, Lu Q, Vieiva S, et al. Incidence and regional distribution of lung overinflation during mechanical ventilation with PEEP. Crit Care Med 2004;32:1496–503.

[39] Tuxen DV. Permissive hypercapneic ventilation. Am J Respir Crit Care Med 1994;150:870–4.

[40] Schultz MJ, Haitsman JJ, Slutsky AS, et al. What tidal volumes should be used in patients without acute lung injury? Anesthesiology 2007;106:1226.

[41] Putensen C, Wrigge H. Tidal volumes in patients with normal lungs. Anesthesiology 2007;106:1085–7.

[42] ACCP/SCCM/AARC Task Force. Evidence based guidelines for weaning and discontinuing mechanical ventilation. Chest 2001;120(6 Suppl):375S–95S.

[43] Cole AGH, Weller SF, Sykes MD. Inverse ratio ventilation compared with PEEP in adult respiratory failure. J Intensive Care Med 1984;10:227–32.

[44] Putensen C, Zech S, Wrigge H, et al. Long term effects of spontaneous breathing during ventilatory

support in patients with ALL. Am J Respir Crit Care
Med 2001;164:43–9.

[45] Varpula T, Valta P, Niemi R, et al. Airway pressure
release ventilation as a primary ventilatory mode in
acute respiratory distress syndrome. Acta Anaesthesiol Scand 2004;48:722–31.

[46] Derdak S, Mehta S, Stewart TE, et al. High-
frequency oscillatory ventilation for acute

respiratory distress syndrome in adults: a randomized. Controlled trial. Am J Respir Crit Care Med
2002;166:801–8.

[47] Available at: www.lshtm.ac.uk/msu/trials/cesar/in
dex.htm. Accessed February 3, 2008.

[48] Rubendeld GD, Cooper C, Carter G, et al. Barriers to
providing lung-protective ventilation to patients with
acute lung injury. Crit Care Med 2004;32:1289–93.

ELSEVIER
SAUNDERS

Clin Chest Med 29 (2008) 233–239

CLINICS IN CHEST MEDICINE

Is There a Best Way to Set Positive Expiratory-End Pressure for Mechanical Ventilatory Support in Acute Lung Injury?

Neil R. MacIntyre, MD

Division of Pulmonary and Critical Care Medicine, Duke University Medical Center,
Box 3911, Room 1120, Erwin Road, Durham, NC 27710, USA

Physiology of alveolar collapse: mechanics and gas exchange

Acute lung injury (ALI) is characterized by airspaces filled with edema fluid, inflammatory cells, and inflammatory cytokines [1–4]. This process is accompanied by surfactant dysfunction and interstitial edema. The end result is loss of airspace gas volume and collapse. Physiologically, this process produces mechanically stiff lung units that have low ventilation/perfusion (V/Q) relationships and shunt. Clinically, ALI is manifest as hypoxemia and the need for high pressures to ventilate the lungs mechanically.

Flooded and collapsed airspaces can be reopened (recruited) when the intra-airspace pressure is raised above the surface tension and extra-airspace pressures produced by lung tissue compliance and thoracic cage mechanical properties [5–10]. Recruitment is usually accomplished by providing positive airway pressure from a mechanical ventilator. The interaction of positive airway pressure and airspace recruitment is complex, however, and involves a number of processes (Fig. 1). First, the positive airway pressure must rise above the critical opening pressure before any gas can enter the airspace. Up to this point, the pressure-volume relationship is flat (ie, there is no volume change over this range of pressures). As pressure above the critical opening pressure is applied, gas is delivered to the airspace to expand it. The pressure-volume relationship becomes steep (ie, substantial volume change occurs as pressure increases). Finally, as airspace expansion

begins to exceed its normal maximal capacity, overstretching occurs and the pressure-volume relationship once again flattens (ie, less volume change occurs because recoil pressures limit further expansion) [8,11,12].

During deflation, the pressure-volume relationships are shifted to the left (ie, less pressure is required for a given airspace gas volume) (see Fig. 1). The major reason for this shift is that during the previous inflation and consequent airspace recruitment, the surfactant monolayer constructs itself to reduce surface tension [13]. Positive end-expiratory pressure (PEEP) can be provided during this deflation to prevent end-expiratory collapse (derecruitment) [5–12]. Specifically, PEEP preserves a certain end-expiratory airspace gas volume and surfactant structure, thereby improving lung mechanical properties and V/Q relationships.

Different regions of an acutely injured lung have different critical opening pressures and pressure-volume relationships because of regional differences in lung injury (ie, regional heterogeneity of airspace pathology) and the gravitational pleural pressure gradient that exists in the lung [7,14–16]. Indeed, in some lung injuries, regions may have no recruitment potential at all [16]. The clinical significance of this is that a given applied airway pressure profile can have differing regional effects. Specifically, an applied airway pressure profile may be inadequate to overcome opening pressure in one region (eg, a severely injured dependent lung unit) but may be excessive in another region (eg, a less-injured nondependent lung region) [7,14–16]. These regional effects produce important clinical challenges, as described below.

E-mail address: neil.macintyre@duke.edu

0272-5231/08/$ - see front matter © 2008 Elsevier Inc. All rights reserved.
doi:10.1016/j.ccm.2008.01.005

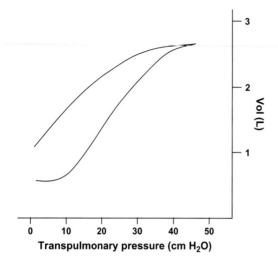

Transpulmonary pressure (cm H_2O)

Fig. 1. Pressure volume relationships in an injured lung
with alveolar collapse. Applying positive pressure (lower
tracing) first adds little volume, as opening pressures
have not been reached. At 10 cm H_2O, recruitment
begins and volume is delivered. At 30 cm H_2O to
35 cm H_2O, the lung is stretched maximally and less volume is delivered. The upper tracing reflects deflation and
is shifted leftward, reflecting better mechanical function.
The lung can remain on the deflation limb with lower
pressures needed for ventilation as long as derecruitment
is prevented with positive end-expiratory pressure.

Repetitive alveolar collapse and expansion
and ventilator-induced lung injury

In experimental animals, ventilator-induced
lung injury (VILI) can be produced by mechanical
ventilation strategies that stretch the lungs beyond
the normal maximum (ie, transpulmonary distending pressures exceeding 30 cm H_2O to 35 cm
H_2O). Pathologically, this overdistension is manifest as diffuse alveolar damage [17–21]. VILI also
seems to occur when injured alveoli are repetitively opened and collapsed during the ventilatory
cycle [17,22,23]. The underlying mechanisms are
thought to involve a shear stress phenomenon in
airspace structures as they suddenly change from
a collapsed state to an inflated state [20]. This
phenomenon may be particularly important at
the interface between adjacent regions that have
differing states of collapse. Shear stress injury
along these interfaces may also occur as a consequence of differing time constants between the
regions.

VILI effects are not restricted to the lungs.
Numerous animal studies have confirmed that an
array of inflammatory cytokines is released into the

systemic circulation as a consequence of VILI [24].
Several clinical studies have indicated that this phenomenon also occurs in mechanically ventilated
patients receiving ventilation at potentially inujuri-
ous settings [25]. Another consequence of VILI
seems to be the loss of the lung's bacterial barrier.
Specifically, several animal studies have shown
that VILI is associated with dramatic increases in
alveolar-capillary bacterial translocation [26].

These systemic effects of VILI may explain
why patients receiving mechanical ventilation for
respiratory failure usually die from multiorgan
failure and shock, not from refractory hypoxemia
or acidemia. It seems that the systemic effects of
VILI, not the lung disease, lead to death. If VILI
could be reduced, mortality might be reduced as
well.

Approaches to attaining and maintaining
alveolar recruitment

Attaining and maintaining alveolar recruitment has three conceptual advantages. First, air
spaces patent throughout the ventilatory cycle
improve gas exchange [1,5,6,27]. Second, avoiding
repetitive alveolar collapse and expansion should
reduce VILI [11,17,22]. Third, air spaces patent
throughout the ventilatory cycle maintain the surfactant monolayer and thus improve the compliance characteristics (ie, lower airway pressures
are required for ventilation as the pressure-
volume relationship is shifted to the left) [5,14].

As noted above, however, critical opening
pressures for different lung regions can cover
a wide range [14,16]. Thus, it may be impossible
to recruit an acutely injured lung fully without
causing overdistension in healthier units. The clinical challenge is thus to provide an overall airway
pressure profile that limits regional overdistension
in the healthiest units and collapse and re-
expansion in the most impaired units [7,8,16].
An additional consideration is balancing the
pressures required for attaining and maintaining
recruitment against the effects of intrathoracic
pressures on cardiac filling and, thus, cardiac
output [28].

Attaining recruitment: tidal breaths
and recruitment maneuvers

Attaining recruitment is a function of lung
inflation. This can be provided with a positive
pressure tidal breath or recruitment maneuvers
(RM). Maintaining recruitment is a function of

PEEP. While tidal breaths may be adequate for appropriate recruitment, RMs should be considered anytime an increase in PEEP is judged necessary for better maintenance of recruitment (or a loss of PEEP from circuit disconnects or if suctioning has occurred). The conceptual goal of an RM is to use a single breath to provide near maximal recruitment and then to bring the lung down on the deflation limb of the pressure-volume curve to the desired level of PEEP [10]. Because the lung is now on the deflation limb, the PEEP to prevent alveolar collapse is generally below the critical opening pressure, and less airway pressure is required for ventilation.

There are several approaches to providing RMs [10,29–32]. First, sigh breaths of 1.5 to 2 times the set tidal volume can be applied every minute or so [29]. Second, the PEEP can be temporarily increased so that the subsequent end-inspiratory volume is raised. Third, the tidal volume can be raised temporarily. Fourth, a high level of continuous positive airway pressure (CPAP) can be applied for a set period of time. The CPAP approach is the most widely reported, probably because it is easy to do and because the RM can be applied for a prolonged time (eg, 30 cm H_2O to 45 cm H_2O CPAP for 30–90 seconds), which may be helpful in recruiting some diseased airspaces.

The response to RMs and the duration of the effect depend heavily on the current mechanical properties of the lung, as well as on the appropriateness of the PEEP setting [10,30–32]. In lungs with minimal recruitment potential (eg, airspaces with inflammation precluding any recruitment or airspaces already recruited), the effect of an RM will be minimal. Conversely, in lungs with high recruitment potential (eg, airspaces with inflammation amenable to positive-pressure opening), the effect of the RM will be substantial. In the latter case, the duration of the effect will depend heavily on the appropriateness of the subsequent PEEP setting with regard to preventing derecruitment [32]. The variability in the literature regarding effectiveness of RMs almost certainly results from these factors.

In general, RMs seem to be safe, although the potential for transient decreases in blood pressure exists. Some patients may require heavy sedation or even paralysis when using RMs of a long duration. There is also the theoretic concern that even relatively short exposures (eg, 15 seconds) to potentially overdistending pressures can cause VILI. Finally, if RMs recruit only airspaces that cannot maintain their patency with the desired level of PEEP, the RMs may contribute to repetitive alveolar collapse and re-expansion.

Inspiratory time manipulations may also help attain recruitment. Indeed, prolonging inspiratory time, generally by adding a pause and often used in conjunction with a rapid decelerating-flow (ie, pressure-targeted) breath, has several physiologic effects. First, the longer inflation period may recruit more slowly recruitable alveoli [33–35]. Second, increased airway-alveolar gas mixing time may improve ventilation-perfusion matching in infiltrative lung disease [33–35]. Third, the development of intrinsic PEEP from short expiratory times can have effects similar to those of applied PEEP (see below) [33]. Fourth, because these long inspiratory times significantly increase total intrathoracic pressures, cardiac output may be affected. Finally, inspiratory to expiratory ratios that exceed 1:1 (so-called inverse ratio ventilation) when applied with older pressure controlled modes are uncomfortable and patient sedation or paralysis may be required.

The development of the pressure release (PR) breath allowing spontaneous breaths to occur during the positive-pressure inflation period has renewed interest in long inspiratory time strategies. A long inspiratory PR breath usually does not require heavy sedation or paralysis because patients can breathe comfortably during mechanical inflation. Proponents also argue that the spontaneous breaths may further enhance lung recruitment and improve cardiac filling [34,35]. This approach was initially termed airway pressure release ventilation (APRV), but it also has received many other colorful names, such as "upside-down synchronized intermittent mechanical ventilation" and "CPAP with release." Although the approach is conceptually appealing, most data for APRV are observational and physiologic in nature [34]. The two small randomized, controlled trials evaluating APRV are inconclusive. One suggested an outcome benefit but had serious design flaws [36,37]; the other showed no outcome benefit [38].

Maintaining recruitment: positive end-expiratory pressure

Given that a tidal breath or RM has recruited the recruitable lung units, what should guide the ultimate PEEP setting to achieve the right balance in optimizing lung recruitment in injured regions while minimizing overdistention in healthier regions? There are visual, mechanical, and gas-exchange approaches to achieving this balance.

In general, the clinical goal is to select a PEEP level that prevents substantial derecruitment throughout the lung (and thus minimizes fraction of inspired oxygen or FiO_2 exposure) without overdistending healthier regions.

With visual approaches, techniques such as computerized tomography (CT) scans provide unparalleled information. Specifically, modern CT scans give detailed analysis of regional lung overdistention, noninjurious ventilation, and fixed and cyclical lung unit collapse (atelectasis) that conceptually are invaluable in assessing mechanical ventilatory support strategies [1,7,8,16]. Unfortunately, CT scans are usually not readily available in intensive care units (ICUs) for routine assessment of ventilator settings. In the future, more readily available visual techniques, such as electrical impedance tomography, breath sound analysis, and radiolabelled gas or aerosol analysis might provide more ICU based visual analyses of lung recruitment and overdistention in critically ill, mechanically ventilated patients [39].

There are several mechanical approaches to assessing recruitment and overdistention. One uses a static pressure-volume plot to set the PEEP/tidal volume combination between the upper and lower inflection points on the deflation limb of the curve [6,11]. A second approach uses step changes in PEEP to determine the level that gives the best compliance [40]. A third uses the pressure profile during a constant flow breath to determine whether recruitment or overdistention is occurring during the tidal breath delivery [41]. With this approach, a concave upward pressure profile reflects overdistention at the end of the breath (excessive PEEP); a convex downward pressure profile reflects recruitment during the breath (inadequate PEEP); and a linear pressure profile suggests no recruitment or overdistention is occurring during the breath (appropriate PEEP). FiO_2 adjustments are then set as low as clinically acceptable. Although conceptually appealing, these mechanical approaches are difficult to perform, often have considerable measurement variability, and have not been subjected to any meaningful clinical outcome studies.

Because of the technical difficulties with the visual and mechanical techniques noted above, gas-exchange criteria are often used clinically to set PEEP. These are generally operationalized as PEEP/FiO_2 tables: tables that dictate stepwise increases or decreases in PEEP/FiO_2 combinations according to some gas-exchange target. Gas-exchange criteria to guide PEEP application are based on the concept that improvements in gas exchange reflect alveolar recruitment [42]. As noted above, however, increased recruitment of very injured lung units may occur only with pressures that injure healthier units. Thus, gas exchange targets today are no longer "maximal" partial pressure of oxygen (PaO_2) values, but rather more modest levels providing adequate oxygenation (eg, PaO_2 55 mm Hg–80 mm Hg). Despite this, constructing a PEEP/FiO_2 table remains an empiric exercise in balancing oxygenation with FiO_2 and lung pressures, and depends on the clinician's perception of the relative "dangers" of high thoracic pressures, high FiO_2, and low PaO_2 [27].

A number of randomized trials over the last decade evaluating different PEEP/FiO_2 tables have provided considerable insight into this process [43–47]. These trials all incorporated a small tidal volume strategy, which in itself likely reduced collapse and reopening injury. These trials generally compared an aggressive versus a conservative PEEP approach. The aggressive PEEP or "open lung" approach stresses recruitment and uses as much PEEP as possible to maximize oxygenation, while usually limiting the PEEP/tidal volume combination to avoid plateau pressure values greater than 30-cm to 35 cm H_2O. The conservative PEEP approach stresses limiting maximal pressures and uses only the minimal amount of PEEP to provide adequate oxygenation with acceptable FiO_2 requirements.

Two of these trials coupled an aggressive PEEP strategy with a small tidal volume strategy and compared that to a high tidal volume/conservative PEEP approach [43,44]. In both trials, the small tidal volume/aggressive PEEP strategy was associated with a lower mortality, but the relative importance of the small tidal volume versus the aggressive PEEP components of the strategy cannot be determined.

Three other large trials used small tidal volumes in all subjects and specifically compared just the PEEP/FiO_2 approaches. The first of these trials was conducted by the Acute Respiratory Distress Syndrome (ARDS) Network [45], and compared its initial PEEP/FiO_2 table to a table that stressed higher PEEP/lower FiO_2 steps (Table 1). The mean day one PEEP in the conservative group was 8 cm H_2O to 9 cm H_2O, as compared with 14 cm H_2O to 15 cm H_2O in the aggressive group. Although the higher PEEP strategy improved lung mechanics, improved oxygenation, and reduced FiO_2 exposure, the study was stopped early because of futility: that is,

Table 1
Two examples of PEEP/FiO$_2$ tables used by the ARDS Network

Conservative approach																
FiO$_2$	.30	.40	.40	.50	.50	.60	.70	.70	.70	.80	.90	.90	.90	1.0	1.0	1.0	1.0
PEEP	5	5	8	8	10	10	10	12	14	14	14	16	18	18	20	22	24
Aggressive approach																
FiO$_2$	.30	.30	.40	.40	.50	.50	.60	.60	.70	.80	.80	.90	1.0	1.0			
PEEP	12	14	14	16	16	18	18	20	20	20	22	22	22	24			

The conservative approach has a minimum of 5 cm H$_2$O PEEP; the aggressive approach has a minimum of 12 cm H$_2$O PEEP. The clinical target is a PO$_2$ of 55 mm Hg–80 mm Hg or oxy-hemoglobin saturation (SpO$_2$) of 88%–95%. If the patient is below these target values, move up the table to the right. If the patient is above these targets, move down the table to the left.

Data from Brower RG, Lanken PN, MacIntyre N, et al. National Heart, Lung, and Blood Institute ARDS Clinical Trials Network. Higher versus lower positive end-expiratory pressures in patients with the acute respiratory distress syndrome. New Engl J Med 2004;351:327–36.

both groups had similar low mortality and a similar duration of mechanical ventilation. There were two concerns about study design, however: one was regarding an imbalance in baseline characteristics favoring the low PEEP group, and one was regarding a change in the high PEEP protocol to raise the minimal level after several hundred subjects had been enrolled. Attempts to statistically account for these issues still failed to find significant differences between the two strategies.

This study was followed by two additional large trials that of this writing have only been reported in abstract format: The Canadian LOVS trial randomized 983 subjects to an aggressive (average PEEP, 16 cm H$_2$O) and a conservative (average PEEP, 10 cm H$_2$O) strategy and demonstrated no outcome difference [46]. The European ExPress trial randomized 850 subjects to an aggressive (PEEP guided by a plateau pressure limit) and a conservative strategy and also demonstrated no mortality difference [47].

Taken together, these trials suggest that in the setting of low tidal volume ventilation, ARDS mortality is consistently low (in the 20%–30% range) and is not affected by the use of either aggressive or conservative PEEP strategies. A criticism of all large trials (including these), however, is that subgroups that might benefit from a specific therapy may not be recognized if they are included in larger numbers of subjects who do not benefit. For example, perhaps patients with good recruitment potential would benefit more to an aggressive PEEP strategy than those without it, or perhaps those with higher VILI risk (eg, high plateau pressures) should be analyzed separately from those with lower risk [7,14–16]. A corollary to this is that the simple PEEP rules used in these trials may not be appropriate in all

patients and that "customized" PEEP approaches should be used [48]. Defining "customization," however, is still much an art form and difficult to study. At the present time, then, all of the PEEP/FiO$_2$ algorithms used in these trials can be considered comparable, easy to use, and as safe and effective as any other strategy reported in the clinical literature.

Summary

Airspace collapse is a hallmark of parenchymal lung injury. Strategies to reopen and maintain patency of these regions offer three advantages: improved gas exchange, less VILI, and improved lung compliance. Elevations in intrathoracic pressure to achieve these goals, however, may overdistend healthier lung regions and compromise cardiac function. PEEP is a widely used technique to maintain alveolar patency, but its beneficial effects must be balanced against its harmful effects. Visual and mechanical approaches to achieve this balance are technically challenging and clinically difficult to do. Gas exchange PEEP/FiO$_2$ algorithms with modest PaO$_2$ goals are as safe and effective as any other strategy reported in the clinical literature.

References

[1] Gattinoni L, Pescenti A, Baglioni S, et al. Inflammatory pulmonary edema and PEEP: correlation between imaging and physiologic studies. J Thorac Imaging 1988;3:59–64.

[2] Pratt PC. Pathology of the adult respiratory distress syndrome. In: Thurlbeck WM, Ael MR, editors. The lung: structure, function and disease. Baltimore (MD): Williams and Wilkins; 1978. p. 43–57.

[3] Fulkerson WJ, Macintyre NR. Pathogenesis and treatment of the adult respiratory distress syndrome. Arch Intern Med 1996;156:29–38.

[4] Ware LB, Matthay MA. The acute respiratory distress syndrome. N Engl J Med 2000;342: 1334–49.

[5] Kacmarek RM, Pierson DJ. AARC Conference on positive end expiratory pressure. Respir Care 1988; 33:419–527.

[6] Kacmarek RM. Strategies to optimize alveolar recruitment. Curr Opin Crit Care 2001;7:15–20.

[7] Gattinoni L, Pelosi P, Crotti S, et al. Effects of positive end expiratory pressure on regional distribution of tidal volume and recruitment in adult respiratory distress syndrome. Am J Respir Crit Care Med 1995;151:1807–14.

[8] Crotti S, Mascheroni D, Caironi P, et al. Recruitment and derecruitment during acute respiratory failure: a clinical study. Am J Respir Crit Care Med 2001;164:131–40.

[9] Hickling KG. Best compliance during a decremental, but not incremental, positive end-expiratory pressure trial is related to open-lung positive end-expiratory pressure: a mathematical model of acute respiratory distress syndrome lungs. Am J Respir Crit Care Med 2001;163:69–78.

[10] Lim SC, Adams AB, Simonson DA, et al. Intercomparison of recruitment maneuver efficacy in three models of acute lung injury. Crit Care Med 2004; 32:2371–7.

[11] Benito S, Lemaire F. Pulmonary pressure-volume relationship in acute respiratory distress syndrome in adults: role of positive end expiratory pressure. J Crit Care 1990;5:27–34.

[12] Putensen C, Bain M, Hormann C. Selecting ventilator settings according to the variables derived from the quasi static pressure volume relationship in patients with acute lung injury. Anesth Analg 1993;77:436–47.

[13] Wyszogrodski I, Kyei-Aboagye K, Taeusch HW Jr, et al. Surfactant inactivation by hyperventilation: conservation by end-expiratory pressure. J Appl Physiol 1975;38:461–6.

[14] Gattinoni L, Caironi P, Pelosi P, et al. What has computed tomography taught us about the acute respiratory distress syndrome? Am J Respir Crit Care Med 2001;164:1701–11.

[15] Thille AW, Richard JC, Maggiore SM, et al. Alveolar recruitment in pulmonary and extrapulmonary acute respiratory distress syndrome: comparison using pressure-volume curve or static compliance. Anesthesiology 2007;106:212–7.

[16] Gattinoni L, Caironi P, Cressoni M, et al. Lung recruitment in patients with the acute respiratory distress syndrome. New Engl J Med 2006;354: 1775–86.

[17] Webb HH, Tierney DF. Experimental pulmonary edema due to intermittent positive pressure ventilation with high inflation pressures: protection by positive end-expiratory pressure. Am Rev Respir Dis 1974;110:556–65.

[18] Dreyfuss D, Savmon G. Ventilator induced lung injury: lessons from experimental studies. Am J Respir Crit Care Med 1998;157:294–323.

[19] Slutsky AS, Ranieri VM. Mechanical ventilation: lessons from the ARDSNet trial. Respir Res 2000; 1:73–7.

[20] Gajic O, Lee J, Doerr CH, et al. Ventilator-induced cell wounding and repair in the intact lung. Am J Respir Crit Care Med 2003;167:1057–63.

[21] Plotz FB, Slutsky AS, van Vught AJ, et al. Ventilator-induced lung injury and multiple system organ failure: a critical review of facts and hypotheses. Intensive Care Med 2004;30:1865–72.

[22] Muscedere JG, Mullen JB, Gan K, et al. Tidal ventilation at low airway pressures can augment lung injury. Am J Respir Crit Care Med 1994;149: 1327–34.

[23] Slutsky AS. Lung injury caused by mechanical ventilation. Chest 1999;116(Suppl 1):9S–15S.

[24] Trembly L, Valenza F, Ribiero SP, et al. Injurious ventilatory strategies increase cytokines and C-fos mRNA expression in an isolated rat lung model. J Clin Invest 1997;99:944–52.

[25] Ranieri VM, Suter PM, Totorella C, et al. Effect of mechanical ventilation on inflammatory mediators in patients with acute respiratory distress syndrome. JAMA 1999;282:54–61.

[26] Nahum A, Hoyt J, Schmitz L, et al. Effect of mechanical ventilation strategy on dissemination of intra-tracheally instilled E-coli in dogs. Crit Care Med 1997;25:1733–43.

[27] Slutsky AS. ACCP Consensus Conference: mechanical ventilation. Chest 1993;104:1833–59.

[28] Pinsky MR, Guimond JG. The effects of positive end-expiratory pressure on heart-lung intcractions. J Crit Care 1991;6:1–15.

[29] Pelosi P, Cadringher P, Bottino N, et al. Sigh in acute respiratory distress syndrome. Am J Respir Crit Care Med 1999;159:872–80.

[30] Rimensberger PC, Prisine G, Mullen BM, et al. Lung recruitment during small tidal volume ventilation allows minimal positive end expiratory pressure without augmenting lung injury. Crit Care Med 1999;27:1940–5.

[31] Grasso S, Mascia L, Del Turco M, et al. Effects of recruiting maneuvers in patients with acute respiratory distress syndrome ventilated with protective ventilatory strategy. Anesthesiology 2002;96(4): 795–802.

[32] Halter JM, Steinberg JM, Schiller HJ, et al. Positive end-expiratory pressure after a recruitment maneuver prevents both alveolar collapse and recruitment/derecruitment. Am J Respir Crit Care Med 2003;167:1620–6.

[33] Cole AGH, Weller SF, Sykes MD. Inverse ratio ventilation compared with PEEP in adult respiratory failure. Intensive Care Med 1984;10:227–32.

[34] Habashi NM. Other approaches to open-lung ventilation: airway pressure release ventilation. Crit Care Med 2005;33(3 Suppl):S228–40.

[35] Stock MC, Downs JB, Frolicher DA. Airway pressure release ventilation. Crit Care Med 1987; 15:462–6.

[36] Putensen C, Zech S, Wrigge H, et al. Long term effects of spontaneous breathing during ventilatory support in patients with ALI. Am J Respir Crit Care Med 2001;164:43–9.

[37] Myers TR, MacIntyre NR. Does airway pressure release ventilation offer important new advantages in mechanical ventilation? Respir Care 2007;52: 452–60.

[38] Varpula T, Valta P, Niemi R, et al. Airway pressure release ventilation as a primary ventilation mode in ARDS. Acta Anaesthesiol Scand 2004; 48:722–31.

[39] Brunow de Carvalho W, Fonseca MC, Johnston C. Electric impedance tomography, the final frontier is close: the bedside reality. Crit Care Med 2007;35: 1996–7.

[40] Suter PM, Fairley HB, Isenberg MD. Optimal end expiratory pressure in patients with acute pulmonary failure. N Engl J Med 1975;292:284–9.

[41] Grasso S, Terragni P, Mascia L, et al. Airway pressure-time curve profile (stress index) detects tidal recruitment/hyperinflation in experimental acute lung injury. Crit Care Med 2004;32:1018–27.

[42] Wagner PD. Ventilation perfusion relationships. Annu Rev Physiol 1980;42:235–47.

[43] Amato MB, Barbas CSV, Medeivos DM, et al. Effect of a protective-ventilation strategy on mortality in the acute respiratory distress syndrome. N Engl J Med 1998;338:347–54.

[44] Villar J, Kacmarek R, Peres-Mendez L, et al. A high positive end expiratory pressure low tidal volume strategy improves outcome in persistent ARDS. Crit Care Med 2006;34:1311–8.

[45] Brower RG, Lanken PN, MacIntyre N, et al. National Heart, Lung, and Blood Institute ARDS Clinical Trials Network. Higher versus lower positive end-expiratory pressures in patients with the acute respiratory distress syndrome. N Engl J Med 2004;351:327–36.

[46] Stewart T, Meade M. LOVS Trial. Presentation at the European Society for Intensive Care Medicine, Barcelona Spain, September 2006.

[47] Mercat A. Express Trial. Presentation at the European Society for Intensive Care Medicine, Barcelona Spain, September 2006.

[48] Marini JJ, Gattinoni L. Ventilatory management of acute respiratory distress syndrome: a consensus of two. Crit Care Med 2004;32:250–5.

ELSEVIER
SAUNDERS

CLINICS
IN CHEST
MEDICINE

Clin Chest Med 29 (2008) 241–252

Protocol-Driven Ventilator Weaning: Reviewing the Evidence

Timothy D. Girard, MD, MSCI[a,*], E. Wesley Ely, MD, MPH[a,b]

[a]Division of Allergy, Pulmonary, and Critical Care Medicine, Center for Health Services Research, Vanderbilt University School of Medicine, 6th Floor MCE, #6110, Nashville, TN 37232-8300, USA
[b]VA Tennessee Valley Geriatric Research, Education and Clinical Center (GRECC), VA Service, Department of Veterans Affairs Medical Center, 1310 24th Avenue South, Nashville, TN 37212-2637, USA

Hundreds of thousands of critically ill patients are mechanically ventilated each year worldwide, and the goal of treatment for each of these patients is expeditious liberation from the ventilator, such that patients breathe without assistance. Delays in this process are associated with significant morbidity, costs, and death. After the inciting cause of respiratory failure has improved, intensive care unit (ICU) practitioners can speed the process leading to successful liberation from the ventilator—classically referred to as "ventilator weaning"—through appropriate management of the ventilator itself. Seminal trials conducted by Brochard and colleagues [1] and Esteban and colleagues [2] in the mid-1990s showed that weaning with synchronized intermittent mandatory ventilation (SIMV) can significantly delay the weaning process. Esteban's trial further identified the spontaneous breathing trial (SBT) as the superior method of weaning. Patients who were managed with SBTs—used to identify their ability to breathe without the assistance of the ventilator—were extubated more quickly than patients who were weaned via gradual reductions in the support provided by intermittent mandatory ventilation (IMV) or pressure support ventilation (PSV).

Only a very small proportion of ICU patients with acute respiratory failure, however, receive treatment during a clinical trial. Thus, for patients to benefit from research findings, such as those established by Tobin, Brochard, Esteban, and many others, the principles that emerge from research studies must be applied in clinical practice, a process that is often delayed and may stall completely [3]. A recent multicenter observational study confirmed that in 349 intensive care units in 23 countries, a large percentage of ICU practitioners continue to employ SIMV weaning, despite strong evidence showing that this method of weaning leads to inferior outcomes. In fact, though the use of daily SBTs rather than SIMV or PSV weaning has been recommended in numerous clinical practice guidelines [4–6] since the publication of Esteban and colleagues' landmark trial over a decade ago, the use of SBTs as a weaning method for patients not extubated after their first trial of spontaneous breathing has actually been decreasing (39% in 1998 versus 28% in 2004, $P<.001$) [7].

Ventilator weaning protocols, by standardizing clinical decision-making, have the potential to greatly improve the translation of research findings into clinical practice, and thereby improve patient outcomes. Typically implemented by respiratory care providers or ICU nurses, weaning protocols have been evaluated by many clinical investigators in the past two decades, but their efficacy and applicability remain a source of controversy. Herein, the authors review the

Dr. Girard receives support from the Hartford Geriatrics Health Outcomes Research Scholars Award Program and the Vanderbilt Physician Scientist Development Program. Dr. Ely receives support from the Veterans Affairs Clinical Science Research and Development Service (VA Merit Review Award) and the National Institutes of Health (AG0727201).

* Corresponding author.
E-mail address: timothy.girard@vanderbilt.edu (T.D. Girard).

rationale and evidence for and against the routine use of weaning protocols, acknowledging from the outset that, having studied weaning protocols as part of their own research [8,9], the authors are not unbiased participants in the debate at hand.

Definitions

A protocol, defined by Merriam-Webster as "a detailed plan of a scientific or medical experiment, treatment, or procedure" [10], may be considered a decision-support tool when used in clinical practice, a tool that lies somewhere between a completely autonomous clinician and a wholly automated computerized treatment in the spectrum of approaches to medical practice (Fig. 1). The appropriate position for a protocol in the spectrum depends on how explicit the protocol is. An "adequately explicit" protocol provides specific rules for decision-making based on patient data [11]. This type of protocol stands in contrast to a practice guideline, which the National Library of Medicine defines as "a set of directions or principles to assist the health care practitioner with patient care decisions about appropriate diagnostic, therapeutic, or other clinical procedures for specific clinical circumstances" [12]. Many practitioners are concerned that practice guidelines represent "cookbook medicine" [13]: that is, an oversimplified approach that is too rigid to apply to individual patients. Unlike practice guidelines, protocols are designed to direct medical treatment in response to data obtained from individual patients. Thus, patients are not all treated the same way; each patient is treated based on their discrete needs, which are expressed through clinical data.

Automated methods of ventilator weaning are now available through the use of computerized, closed loop ventilator systems. Automation lies at the opposite end of the spectrum from the autonomous clinician, because the weaning process occurs by itself with little or no direct human control. Most of the weaning protocol studies conducted to date have compared protocols implemented by nonphysician health care professionals to traditional physician-directed weaning, but a few trials have examined the efficacy of computerized weaning strategies.

Rationale supporting the use of weaning protocols

As listed in Box 1, proponents of weaning protocols endorse the use of protocols for reasons that can be divided into two categories: the variability and ineffectiveness of physician-directed weaning, and the efficacy and efficiency of weaning protocols.

The modern practice of medicine, though marked by relentless progress and responsible for the greatly improved health enjoyed by recent generations, continues to be characterized by variability and error when compared with other industries [14]. Intensive care medicine is no exception, and physician-directed approaches to ventilator weaning vary widely from ICU to ICU and from physician to physician. As stated previously, Esteban and colleagues [7] recently determined that daily SBTs are infrequently used in the management of patients not extubated after their first trial of spontaneous breathing. Additionally, when the investigators compared mechanical ventilation practices in an international 2004 cohort of 1,675 subjects to a 1998 cohort of 1,383 subjects, they observed that SIMV weaning continues to be used despite this method's proven association with inferior outcomes; one out of every six subjects in the 2004 cohort was weaned using SIMV (Table 1). Unfortunately, these data (along with a large body of evidence; see Refs. [15–18]) strongly suggest that it is not true in general that "physicians are adept at extracting principles that emerge from research studies and incorporating them into their everyday practice" [19].

In the ICU, numerous factors contribute to variability in practice and deviations from the method of weaning proven to result in superior outcomes, and protocols have been promoted because of their relative immunity to these factors. First, physician-directed weaning is often guided

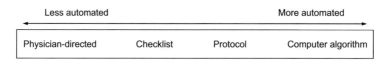

Fig. 1. Spectrum of approaches to ventilator weaning.

Box 1. Rationale supporting the use of weaning protocols

Less limited and biased by human decision-making than physician-directed weaning

Developed based on best evidence; less influenced by personal or local opinion

Efficacy and safety supported by numerous clinical investigations

Can make up for limitations in local resources or staff availability

Free physicians to perform other duties in the ICU

Facilitate quality monitoring and improvement

Can be the basis of a systematic approach to learning

Enhance transparency and communication

by local opinion and local supply of resources rather than by science [15]. Protocols, alternatively, provide a link between research findings and clinical practice; their use reduces unwanted variability in practice by stabilizing the decision-making process. Second, even experienced ICU practitioners have a limited capacity to store and process information [20], and complexities encountered during the management of a critically ill patient can quickly exceed this capacity. In addition, ICU physicians are susceptible to cognitive biases—including omission bias and status quo bias—that may adversely affect decision-making

Table 1
Comparison of methods used during ventilator weaning according to two multicenter, international, prospective cohort investigations

Weaning method, %	1998 cohort	2004 cohort	P value
SIMV	11	1.6	<0.001
SIMV+PSV	26	15	<0.001
PSV	19	55	<0.001
Daily SBT	39	27.7	<0.001
Not reported (NR)	5	0.7	NR

Esteban and colleagues [7] determined the methods used to wean patients not extubated after the first attempt of spontaneous breathing during two large cohort investigations, and found the percentage of patients weaned with daily SBTs has fallen, while the percentage weaned with PSV has significantly increased.

[21]. These limitations and biases may, in part, explain physicians' failure to identify some patients who are ready for extubation, a fact evidenced by studies showing that only 50% of patients who self-extubate require reintubation [22]. Of course, this shortcoming on the part of physicians may also result from the low-intensity physician staffing patterns that characterize many ICUs [23]. When faced with the responsibility of managing the care of a large number of critically ill patients, most physicians focus their efforts on the unstable patients; stable patients, such as those in the weaning period, may receive less attention. Through the use of weaning protocols, ICU physicians can ensure that stable patients are managed consistently during the weaning period and that decisions regarding their weaning are less likely to be influenced by the limitations and biases that affect human decision-making. While the use of protocols actively improves the management of patients being weaned, proponents contend that the care of unstable patients may be improved as well because physicians are free to perform duties that cannot be delegated to others.

The efficacy of weaning protocols (implemented by either nonphysician health care professionals or by computers) has been compared with that of physician-directed weaning in multiple clinical investigations, which the authors will review in more detail. Proponents point to the fact that the majority of these investigations concluded that weaning protocols lead to superior outcomes, compared with physician-directed weaning (Table 2). One trial, however, suggested that physician-directed weaning is superior, and an important minority showed no difference in outcomes. In addition to the improvement in clinical outcomes observed in many trials for patients managed with weaning protocols, protocols may improve efficiency in ICUs and provide other benefits, though these purported benefits have not been studied. First, the use of protocols provides a means by which quality can be measured; adherence to a protocol can be tracked and analyzed, whereas decisions made during physician-directed weaning cannot be tracked and classified as correct or erroneous with reliability. Moreover, objections to or deviations from the directions of an explicit protocol—objections that are ideally based on scientific evidence—can be documented to provide the basis of developing better protocols: that is, serve as the basis of a systematic approach to learning [24]. Finally, protocols may serve to inform patients and their families

Table 2
Studies comparing weaning protocols to physician-directed weaning

Reference	n	Patient population[a]	Outcomes improved by protocol
Studies favoring weaning protocols			
Randomized controlled trials			
Ely et al, 1996 [8]	300	Medical and cardiac	Ventilator time, ICU costs, complications
Kollef et al, 1997 [37]	357	Medical and surgical	Ventilator time[b]
Marelich et al, 2000 [31]	385	Medical and trauma	Ventilator time[b]
Schultz et al, 2001 [35]	223	Pediatric	Weaning time[b]
Lellouche et al, 2006 [52]	144	Medical and surgical	Ventilator time, ICU LOS
Girard et al, 2008 [9]	336	Medical	Ventilator time, ICU and hospital LOS, survival
Cohort studies			
Foster et al, 1984 [27]	63	Cardiac surgery	Ventilator time
Wood et al, 1995 [28]	284	Cardiac surgery	Ventilator time
Saura et al, 1996 [39]	101	Medical	Ventilator time, ICU LOS
Horst et al, 1998 [40]	893	Surgical	Ventilator time[b]
Scheinhorn et al, [41]	490	Long-term acute-care	Weaning time, hospital LOS
Vitacca et al, 2001[c] [42]	52	Long-term acute-care	Ventilator time, LWU and hospital LOS
Smyrnios et al, 2002 [43]	734	Medical and surgical	Ventilator time, ICU and hospital LOS, costs
Grap et al, 2003 [44]	928	Medical	Ventilator time
Dries et al, 2004 [45]	650	Surgical	Ventilator time, VAP[b]
Restrepo et al, 2004 [46]	187	Pediatric	Weaning time
Bumroongkit et al, 2005 [47]	394	Medical	Ventilator time, ICU LOS
Tonnelier et al, 2005 [48]	208	Medical and surgical	Ventilator time, ICU LOS[b]
Aboutanos et al, 2006 [49]	69	Trauma	Ventilator time
Studies showing no difference			
Randomized controlled trials			
McKinley et al, 2001 [32]	67	Trauma	None
Namen et al, 2001 [34]	100	Neurosurgical	None
Randolph et al, 2002 [36]	182	Pediatric	None
Cohort studies			
Djunaedi et al, 1997 [56]	107	Medical and surgical	None
Duane et al, 2002 [33]	328	Trauma	None
Krishnan et al, 2004 [38]	299	Medical	None
Studies favoring physician-directed weaning			
Cohort studies			
Blackwood et al, 2006 [50]	411	Medical and surgical	None improved, but ICU LOS worsened

　　Pilot studies that were not powered to detect differences in outcomes are not shown.
　　Abbreviations: LOS, length of stay; LWU, long-term weaning unit; VAP, ventilator-associated pneumonia.
　　[a] Only adults were enrolled unless otherwise noted.
　　[b] Stratified analyses suggested that the weaning protocol was beneficial for some patients but did not improve outcomes for other patients, compared with physician-directed weaning.
　　[c] All patients in a randomized trial of two weaning protocols were compared with controls managed by physician-directed weaning.

regarding the treatment plan during weaning [25]. Documented protocols, as well as other decision-support tools such as practice guidelines and checklists, can be disseminated as needed to improve communication in the ICU between health care providers and patients or family members and between various members of the health care team.

Concerns about the use of weaning protocols

　　Criticisms of the routine use of weaning protocols typically consist of direct responses to the rationale supporting the use of protocols, calling attention to the effectiveness and flexibility of physician-directed weaning and the inconsistencies in research findings regarding the efficacy of weaning protocols (Box 2). Additionally, some have raised concerns about the effects of protocols on medical education and have suggested that the efficacy of alternative decision-support tools and superior ICU design strategies make weaning protocols unnecessary.

Modern medicine continues a long-held tradition of heavy reliance on well-trained and highly skilled physicians, and many critics of weaning protocols agree with the assertion that "an intelligent physician who customizes knowledge generated by a previous research protocol to the particulars of each patient is expected to outperform the inflexible application of [a weaning] protocol" [19]. Because every patient is unique, protocols are considered by many to be incapable of recognizing the specific needs of an individual patient and adapting the treatment plan appropriately in response to these needs. Physicians, on the other hand, have great potential when evaluating an individual patient; not only can they respond to unique problems that arise during weaning, but innovations in practice that improve outcomes may be discovered by the astute clinician. This assumes, of course, that such innovations result in improvements that are dramatic enough to be recognized, and most purposeful clinical interventions have relatively small effects that cannot be recognized apart from the analyses conducted as part of systematic clinical research [11].

Box 2. Rationale supporting the use of physician-directed weaning

Flexible and adaptive to the needs of individual patients

Can lead to innovative changes in practice

Equivalent to weaning protocols in some studies, especially in ICUs with high staffing levels

Promotes education and leads to highly skilled practitioners

Does not require the additional resources needed to design, implement, and sustain weaning protocol use

Avoids institution-wide acceptance of a treatment strategy before best evidence is available

---

Investigations that have compared weaning protocols to physician-directed weaning, whether randomized, controlled trials or prospective cohort studies, have yielded varying results (see Table 2); this has been interpreted by critics of weaning protocols as a lack of evidence to support the efficacy of weaning protocols. In general, when protocols are implemented before the treatments they promote are rigorously proven efficacious in well-designed clinical trials, unproven therapies may become propagated and institutionalized prematurely, such that they are difficult to rescind or even study in a randomized fashion [24]. The heterogeneous results of weaning protocol trials suggest that additional research is needed, especially among patient populations in which protocols have not been studied and in ICUs that use new design strategies and technologies that might diminish the need for weaning protocols. The dogmatic application of protocols in such environments may hinder future research and progress.

Much of medical education consists of on-the-job training, and critics of weaning protocols have raised concerns that their use will impair education and lead to deskilled practitioners who are poorly equipped to handle the variations between the patients they will encounter. In fact, some have projected that the use of protocols may facilitate the replacement of physicians with less expensive, less skilled workers who may be incapable of operating effectively in diverse situations. The viewpoint that expert physicians possess special and ineffable wisdom that cannot be translated into a protocol, however, may significantly interfere with the education of young physicians by excusing the experts from the challenge of articulating precisely how decisions should be made [11]. Though some research exists regarding medical education and critical care, the effects of protocols on the development of trainees are not well documented.

The impact of intensivists, closed ICUs, and regionalization of intensive care to high-volume hospitals on ICU outcomes has recently received much attention [26], and these changes in the delivery of intensive care—as well as the use of other decision-support tools, such as checklists—may significantly influence the value of weaning protocols in some ICUs. Specifically, a closed ICU that has a high level of staffing by intensivists who use weaning checklists may see no improvement in outcomes with the implementation of a weaning protocol. The corollary to this supposition, of course, is that an open ICU with a low level of staffing of nonintensivists who do not use weaning checklists would likely greatly improve outcomes by using a weaning protocol. This ICU, like any ICU that uses protocols, would need to design the protocol, implement and promote it, and sustain its use, and critics contend that a significant amount of resources are required for this process to be successful.

Reviewing the evidence

The earliest investigations of the efficacy of weaning protocols were conducted in surgical ICUs, where it was found that respiratory therapist-driven protocols—perhaps most appropriately referred to as extubation protocols—resulted in earlier extubation for uncomplicated postoperative cardiac surgery patients, compared with management by physicians [27,28]. Though these studies suggested that nonphysician health care professionals can effectively manage the weaning process using protocols, the influence of these studies was limited by the homogeneous patient populations enrolled and the lack of a randomized study design.

In 1996, recognizing that physicians often do not discontinue mechanical ventilation expeditiously despite advances in weaning methodology [1,2], Ely and coworkers [8] conducted the first randomized, controlled trial to compare a weaning protocol driven by nonphysician health care professionals to traditional physician-directed weaning. The 151 medical and coronary ICU subjects who were managed with a two-step protocol involving a daily weaning screen followed by an SBT (when patients passed the screen) were liberated from mechanical ventilation 1.5 days earlier than the 149 subjects managed with physician-directed weaning (median duration of mechanical ventilation, 4.5 versus 6 days; $P = .003$) (Fig. 2). In addition, the weaning protocol resulted in lower median ICU costs ($15,740 versus $20,890, $P = .03$) and fewer complications of respiratory failure (20% versus 41%, $P = .001$).

Critics have suggested that these results are invalid, claiming that the study design resulted in a high percentage of subjects in the control group being managed with IMV after enrollment, whereas subjects in the protocol group were managed with daily SBTs: "To conclude that protocols are superior, weaning methods need to be the same in the protocol and usual-care arms" [29]. In clinical research, randomization aims to create groups of participants that do not differ, except with respect to the intervention [30]. In the trial in question, in fact, the number of subjects managed with IMV or IMV plus PSV before enrollment was similar in the intervention and control groups (71% versus 76%). Use of IMV after

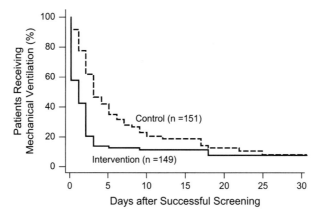

Fig. 2. Effect of a weaning protocol on the duration of mechanical ventilation in medical ICU patients with acute respiratory failure. The weaning protocol consisted of a daily screen of respiratory function followed by a 2-hour spontaneous breathing trial in those who met the screening criteria. After adjustment for the severity of illness at baseline, as measured by the acute physiology and chronic health evaluation (APACHE II) score, age, sex, race, location of the ICU, and duration of intubation before enrollment, a Cox proportional-hazards analysis showed that mechanical ventilation was discontinued more rapidly in the intervention group than in the control group (relative risk of successful extubation, 2.13; 95% confidence index or CI, 1.55 to 2.92; $P < .001$). (*From* Ely EW, Baker AM, Dunagan DP, et al. Effect on the duration of mechanical ventilation of identifying patients capable of breathing spontaneously. N Engl J Med 1996;335(25):1866; with permission. Copyright © 1996, Massachusetts Medical Society.)

enrollment, however, was not mandated by study design: "Neither the mode of ventilation nor the weaning strategy used [in the control group] was specified" [8]. Thus, any differences in the management of subjects in the intervention versus control groups resulted from the practice habits and beliefs of the ICU physicians managing subjects in the control group. The fact that these habits and beliefs are often inconsistent with the best available evidence is the basis of arguments in favor of the use of weaning protocols.

Numerous investigations have been conducted since Ely and colleagues' study was published a decade ago, and results have varied depending on the patient population studied (see Table 2). Marelich and colleagues [31], for example, randomized 385 medical and trauma ICU subjects to a weaning protocol consisting of a daily screen followed by SBTs when appropriate, or to physician-directed weaning, and found that the weaning protocol significantly reduced the duration of mechanical ventilation ($P = .0001$). A stratified analysis suggested that the greatest benefit was realized by medical, rather than trauma, ICU subjects. These findings are consistent with those of Ely and colleagues, who observed a benefit among medical ICU patients, as well as those of McKinley and colleagues [32], who conducted a randomized controlled trial among a homogeneous population of 67 trauma ICU subjects and found that a computer-driven weaning protocol resulted in outcomes similar to physician-directed weaning.

Another large study of weaning protocols in a trauma population yielded results similar to those of McKinley and colleagues. In a prospective cohort study of 328 trauma ICU subjects, Duane and colleagues [33] observed no improvement in outcomes attributable to weaning protocols. Neurosurgical patients represent another population in which studies of weaning protocols have yielded negative results. Namen and colleagues [34] conducted the only randomized, controlled trial of a weaning protocol in a neurosurgical population and observed similar outcomes in the two treatment groups. Mental status—which was significantly depressed in a large number of subjects—was independently associated with extubation outcome ($P = .0006$), leading the investigators to conclude that a weaning protocol based on traditional parameters of respiratory physiology is of limited use in the management of neurosurgical patients [34].

Two randomized, controlled trials that evaluated the efficacy of weaning protocols in pediatric ICUs yielded different results. Schultz and colleagues [35] randomized 223 children in pediatric and coronary ICUs to management with a weaning protocol or physician-directed weaning; weaning time was significantly reduced for those managed with a weaning protocol (median weaning time, 10 versus 0.8 hours; $P < .001$). Total duration of mechanical ventilation was not significantly reduced (median ventilator time, 27.5 versus 23.8 hours; $P = .26$), but this may be because of the high percentage of patients with nonrespiratory indications for intubation. The improvement in weaning time was more pronounced among subjects with a respiratory indication for intubation and ventilation (median weaning time, 56.1 versus 3.8 hours; $P = .01$) than among those with nonrespiratory indications (median weaning time, 4.1 versus 0.7 hours; $P < .001$). Based on these results, the pediatric subjects randomized by Randolph and colleagues [36] to protocol-directed weaning would be expected to have superior outcomes because the majority had respiratory indications for intubation. The trial found no significant differences in outcomes between treatment groups, but compliance with the weaning protocols was maintained for only 66% of subjects randomized to weaning protocols. As observed in the trial of neurosurgical subjects, mental status was associated with the likelihood of extubation; management of respiratory function alone via a weaning protocol was insufficient to improve outcomes.

Trials conducted by Kollef and colleagues [37] and Krishnan and colleagues [38] suggest that existing ICU practices and staffing patterns are important determinants of whether weaning protocols will be of benefit. Kollef and colleagues [37] randomized 357 medical and surgical subjects in four separate ICUs to protocol-directed or physician-directed weaning. Though protocol-directed weaning lead to earlier extubation in the population as a whole, and stratified analyses of results within ICUs were underpowered, the results suggested that the weaning protocol had no benefit in the ICU in which nursing-directed weaning was part of the culture [37].

Krishnan and colleagues [38] conducted a nonrandomized prospective trial in a closed medical ICU characterized by high intensivist staffing levels and structured rounds during which a weaning checklist was used each day. In this setting, a weaning protocol did not improve the outcomes when compared with usual care. Taken together with the trials conducted by Ely and colleagues

[8] and Marelich and colleagues [31], as well as numerous prospective cohort studies that have found weaning protocols to be beneficial [39–49], the authors conclude that most medical and surgical ICUs that do not have the level of staffing reported by Krishnan and coworkers (9.5 physician-hours per bed per day, Ref. [38]), and do not use some form of decision-support tool regarding weaning, can significantly improve outcomes through the use of a weaning protocol. In fact, only one study to date has reported inferior outcomes among patients managed with weaning protocols. In a nonrandomized prospective study, Blackwood and colleagues [50] found that ICU length of stay was longer for subjects in phase II (after a weaning protocol was implemented) than for patients in phase I (preweaning protocol). This result was because of an increase in the time from extubation to ICU discharge, a period that should not have been influenced by a weaning protocol, and no obvious reason for this change was identified.

Computer-driven weaning protocols were being studied nearly two decades ago, when Strickland and Hasson [51] found that a computer-controlled weaning system significantly reduced time to wean in a 15-subject pilot investigation. The promise of computer-driven weaning was recently confirmed in a large randomized trial conducted by Lellouche and colleagues [52]. In a multicenter trial that enrolled 144 medical and surgical ICU subjects, those managed with a closed-loop computerized system that drives PSV in response to real time clinical data had significantly shorter ventilator and ICU stays than subjects in the control group. Physician-controlled weaning was conducted according to the practice in local ICUs, where weaning guidelines were readily available. The investigators estimated, though, that adherence to guidelines was modest: SBTs were performed during only half of all days when ventilator parameters should have prompted a trial [52].

As described previously, trials conducted by Namen and colleagues [34] and Randolph and colleagues [36] found that weaning protocols that do not address level of consciousness may be ineffective in some ICUs. The effect of mental status as well as sedation strategy [53] on duration of mechanical ventilation and other important outcomes led several investigators to study the efficacy of protocol-driven sedation in ICU patients. Brook and colleagues [54] randomized 321 mechanically ventilated medical ICU subjects to sedation per usual care or management with a sedation protocol that emphasized use of intermittent bolus, rather than infusions, to maintain a sedation target specified via a validated sedation

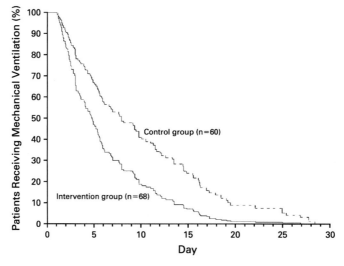

Fig. 3. Effect of daily interruption of sedative infusions on the duration of mechanical ventilation in medical ICU patients receiving sedatives. After adjustment for age, sex, weight, APACHE II score, and type of respiratory failure, mechanical ventilation was discontinued earlier in the intervention group than in the control group (relative risk of extubation, 1.9; 95% CI, 1.3 to 2.7; $P < .001$). (*From* Kress JP, Pohlman AS, O'Connor MF, et al. Daily interruption of sedative infusions in critically ill patients undergoing mechanical ventilation. N Engl J Med 2000;342(20):1474; with permission. Copyright © 2000, Massachusetts Medical Society.)

Box 3. "Wake up and breathe" protocol

Spontaneous awakening trial safety screen
If the patient has no evidence of the following criteria, proceed with SAT. Otherwise, reassess the next day.
Active seizures or alcohol withdrawal requiring a sedative infusion
Ongoing agitation requiring escalating sedative doses
Active treatment with neuromuscular blockers
Myocardial ischemia in the previous 24 hours
Increased intracranial pressure

Spontaneous awakening trial
Discontinue sedatives and analgesics used for sedation and monitor for the following failure criteria. If observed, restart sedatives at half the previous dose, titrate to achieve patient comfort, and restart protocol the next day.
Sustained anxiety, agitation, or pain.
Respiratory rate greater than 35/min for at least 5 minutes
SpO_2 less than 88% for at least 5 minutes
Acute cardiac dysrhythmia
Two or more signs of respiratory distress, including tachycardia, bradycardia, accessory muscle use, abdominal paradox, diaphoresis, or marked dyspnea

Spontaneous breathing trial safety screen
If the patient passes the SAT and has no evidence of the following criteria, proceed with SBT. Otherwise, reassess the next day.
SpO_2 less than 88% or FiO_2 greater than 50% or PEEP greater than 8 cm H_2O
Lack of spontaneous inspiratory efforts
Agitation
Myocardial ischemia in the previous 24 hours
Dopamine or dobutamine greater than or equal to 5 µg/kg per minute, norepinephrine greater than or equal to 2 µg/min, or any vasopressin or milrinone at any dose
Increased intracranial pressure

Spontaneous breathing trial
Discontinue ventilatory support, placing patient on T-piece or PSV less than 8 cm H_2O, and monitor for the following criteria. If observed, restart full support using previous ventilator settings, titrate as needed, and restart protocol the next day.
Respiratory rate greater than 35/min or less than 8/min for at least 5 minutes
SpO_2 less than 88% for at least 5 minutes
Abrupt changes in mental status
Acute cardiac dysrhythmia
Two or more signs of respiratory distress, including tachycardia, bradycardia, accessory muscle use, abdominal paradox, diaphoresis, or marked dyspnea
If the patient does not develop any failure criteria during a 120-min trial, consider extubation.

Abbreviations: FiO_2, fraction of inspired oxygen; PEEP, positive end-expiratory pressure; PSV, pressure support ventilation; SAT, spontaneous awakening trial; SBT, spontaneous awakening trial; SpO_2, oxygen saturation.

---

scale. Compared with those in the control group, subjects in the sedation protocol group had a shorter duration of mechanical ventilation (median, 55.9 versus 117 hours; $P = .008$) as well as shorter ICU and hospital stays. Kress and colleagues [55] refined their approach to sedation in a different way by developing a protocol that paralleled the approach to weaning taken by Ely and

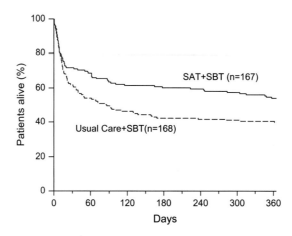

Fig. 4. Effect of paired sedation and ventilator weaning protocol on one-year survival in medical ICU patients receiving mechanical ventilation. An unadjusted Cox proportional-hazard analysis showed that patients in the SAT plus SBT group were 32% less likely to die at any instant during the year following enrollment than patients in the usual care plus SBT group (hazard ratio for death, 0.68; 95% CI, 0.50 to 0.92; $P = .01$). (*Reprinted from* Girard TD, Kress JP, Fuchs BD, et al. Efficacy and safety of a paired sedation and ventilator weaning protocol for mechanically ventilated patients in intensive care (Awakening and Breathing Controlled trial): a randomized controlled trial. Lancet 2008;371(9607):131; with permission.)

colleagues. Patients were screened each day and for those who passed the screen, sedation was interrupted (similar to interruption of mechanical ventilation during an SBT). In a randomized, controlled trial that enrolled 128 mechanically ventilated medical ICU subjects, those managed with daily interruption of sedatives had a shorter duration of mechanical ventilation (median, 4.9 versus 7.3 days; $P = .004$) (Fig. 3) and shorter ICU stays than subjects in the control group.

In light of this evidence, any approach to weaning must consider level of consciousness and sedation status in addition to respiratory function and mechanical ventilator settings. Thus, the authors expanded the scope of the traditional weaning protocol. The "wake up and breathe" protocol includes an evaluation of sedation status and a spontaneous awakening trial (SAT), which are paired with a weaning screen and an SBT (Box 3). In a multicenter randomized trial that enrolled 335 medical ICU subjects, the authors found that the paired "wake up and breathe" protocol dramatically improves outcomes, such that subjects managed with a paired SAT plus SBT protocol spent more days breathing without assistance than did those managed with sedation per usual care and a ventilator weaning protocol consisting of daily SBTs (14.7 versus 11.6 days during the 28-day study period; mean difference, 3.1 days, 95% CI, 0.7 to 5.6; $P = .02$) [9]. Additionally, subjects in the SAT

plus SBT group were discharged from the ICU (median ICU stay, 9.1 versus 12.9 days; $P = .01$) and hospital (median hospital stay, 14.9 versus 19.2 days; $P = .04$) earlier, and they were less likely to die in the year following enrollment than were subjects in the control group (hazard ratio for death, 0.68; 95% CI, 0.50 to 0.92; $P = .01$) (Fig. 4), confirming that incremental improvements in outcomes are achieved through the protocol-driven management of sedation and ventilator weaning.

Summary

Protocol-driven ventilator weaning has the potential to improve clinical outcomes by increasing the use of efficacious weaning methods, such as daily weaning screens and spontaneous breathing trials, and the recently-studied "wake up and breathe" protocol represents a new generation of weaning that pairs management of the ventilator and sedation to achieve superior outcomes. Clinical trials have demonstrated that weaning protocols—whether driven by nonphysician health care professionals or closed-loop computer systems—can reduce the duration of mechanical ventilation and lead to earlier ICU and hospital discharge in many ICUs. The benefits of weaning protocols, however, may not be universal, and factors such as patient population, ICU design and staffing, and use of other decision-support tools must be considered when deciding where and how to implement protocols.

References

[1] Brochard L, Rauss A, Benito S, et al. Comparison of three methods of gradual withdrawal from ventilatory support during weaning from mechanical ventilation. Am J Respir Crit Care Med 1994;150(4): 896–903.

[2] Esteban A, Frutos F, Tobin MJ, et al. A comparison of four methods of weaning patients from mechanical ventilation. Spanish Lung Failure Collaborative Group. N Engl J Med 1995;332(6):345–50.

[3] Lenfant C. Shattuck lecture—clinical research to clinical practice—lost in translation? N Engl J Med 2003;349(9):868–74.

[4] MacIntyre NR, Cook DJ, Ely EW Jr, et al. Evidence-based guidelines for weaning and discontinuing ventilatory support: a collective task force facilitated by the American College of Chest Physicians; the American Association for Respiratory Care; and the American College of Critical Care Medicine. Chest 2001;120(6 Suppl):375S–95S.

[5] Boles JM, Bion J, Connors A, et al. Weaning from mechanical ventilation. Eur Respir J 2007;29(5): 1033–56.

[6] Dellinger RP, Levy MM, Carlet JM, et al. Surviving Sepsis Campaign: International guidelines for management of severe sepsis and septic shock: 2008. Intensive Care Med 2007;34(1):17–60.

[7] Esteban A, Ferguson ND, Meade MO, et al. Evolution of mechanical ventilation in response to clinical research. Am J Respir Crit Care Med 2008;177(2): 170–7.

[8] Ely EW, Baker AM, Dunagan DP, et al. Effect on the duration of mechanical ventilation of identifying patients capable of breathing spontaneously. N Engl J Med 1996;335(25):1864–9.

[9] Girard TD, Kress JP, Fuchs BD, et al. Efficacy and safety of a paired sedation and ventilator weaning protocol for mechanically ventilated patients in intensive care (Awakening and Breathing Controlled trial): a randomised controlled trial. Lancet 2008; 371(9607):126–34.

[10] Merriam-Webster Online: protocol. Available at: http://www.merriam-webster.com/dictionary/protocol. Accessed February 15, 2008.

[11] Morris AH. Rational use of computerized protocols in the intensive care unit. Crit Care 2001;5(5): 249–54.

[12] National Library of Medicine–medical subject headings: practice guideline. Available at: http://www. nlm.nih.gov/cgi/mesh/2008/MB_cgi?mode=&term= PRACTICE+GUIDELINE. Accessed February 15, 2008.

[13] Tunis SR, Hayward RS, Wilson MC, et al. Internists' attitudes about clinical practice guidelines. Ann Intern Med 1994;120(11):956–63.

[14] Kohn LT, Corrigan JM, Donaldson MS, editors. To err is human: building a safer health system. Washington, DC: National Academy Press; 2000.

[15] Wennberg JE. Unwarranted variations in healthcare delivery: implications for academic medical centres. BMJ 2002;325(7370):961–4.

[16] Grol R, Grimshaw J. From best evidence to best practice: effective implementation of change in patients' care. Lancet 2003;362(9391):1225–30.

[17] Berenholtz S, Pronovost PJ. Barriers to translating evidence into practice. Curr Opin Crit Care 2003; 9(4):321–5.

[18] Ilan R, Fowler RA, Geerts R, et al. Knowledge translation in critical care: factors associated with prescription of commonly recommended best practices for critically ill patients. Crit Care Med 2007; 35(7):1696–702.

[19] Tobin MJ. Of principles and protocols and weaning. Am J Respir Crit Care Med 2004;169(6):661–2.

[20] Cowan N. The magical number 4 in short-term memory: a reconsideration of mental storage capacity. Behav Brain Sci 2001;24(1):87–114.

[21] Aberegg SK, Haponik EF, Terry PB. Omission bias and decision making in pulmonary and critical care medicine. Chest 2005;128(3):1497–505.

[22] Mion LC, Minnick AF, Leipzig R, et al. Patient-initiated device removal in intensive care units: a national prevalence study. Crit Care Med 2007; 35(12):2714–20.

[23] Pronovost PJ, Angus DC, Dorman T, et al. Physician staffing patterns and clinical outcomes in critically ill patients: a systematic review. JAMA 2002; 288(17):2151–62.

[24] Chatburn RL, Deem S. Should weaning protocols be used with all patients who receive mechanical ventilation? Respir Care 2007;52(5):609–19.

[25] Timmermans S, Mauck A. The promises and pitfalls of evidence-based medicine. Health Aff (Millwood) 2005;24(1):18–28.

[26] Kahn JM, Brake H, Steinberg KP. Intensivist physician staffing and the process of care in academic medical centres. Qual Saf Health Care 2007;16(5): 329–33.

[27] Foster GH, Conway WA, Pamulkov N, et al. Early extubation after coronary artery bypass: brief report. Crit Care Med 1984;12(11):994–6.

[28] Wood G, MacLeod B, Moffatt S. Weaning from mechanical ventilation: physician-directed vs a respiratory-therapist-directed protocol. Respir Care 1995; 40(3):219–24.

[29] Tobin MJ. Remembrance of weaning past: the seminal papers. Intensive Care Med 2006;32(10):1485–93.

[30] Moher D, Schulz KF, Altman DG. The CONSORT statement: revised recommendations for improving the quality of reports of parallel-group randomized trials. Ann Intern Med 2001;134(8):657–62.

[31] Marelich GP, Murin S, Battistella F, et al. Protocol weaning of mechanical ventilation in medical and surgical patients by respiratory care practitioners

and nurses: effect on weaning time and incidence of ventilator-associated pneumonia. Chest 2000; 118(2):459–67.

[32] McKinley BA, Moore FA, Sailors RM, et al. Computerized decision support for mechanical ventilation of trauma induced ARDS: results of a randomized clinical trial. J Trauma 2001;50(3): 415–24.

[33] Duane TM, Riblet JL, Golay D, et al. Protocol-driven ventilator management in a trauma intensive care unit population. Arch Surg 2002;137(11): 1223–7.

[34] Namen AM, Ely EW, Tatter SB, et al. Predictors of successful extubation in neurosurgical patients. Am J Respir Crit Care Med 2001;163(3 Pt 1): 658–64.

[35] Schultz TR, Lin RJ, Watzman HM, et al. Weaning children from mechanical ventilation: a prospective randomized trial of protocol-directed versus physician-directed weaning. Respir Care 2001;46(8): 772–82.

[36] Randolph AG, Wypij D, Venkataraman ST, et al. Effect of mechanical ventilator weaning protocols on respiratory outcomes in infants and children: a randomized controlled trial. JAMA 2002;288(20): 2561–8.

[37] Kollef MH, Shapiro SD, Silver P, et al. A randomized, controlled trial of protocol-directed versus physician-directed weaning from mechanical ventilation. Crit Care Med 1997;25(4):567–74.

[38] Krishnan JA, Moore D, Robeson C, et al. A prospective, controlled trial of a protocol-based strategy to discontinue mechanical ventilation. Am J Respir Crit Care Med 2004;169(6):673–8.

[39] Saura P, Blanch L, Mestre J, et al. Clinical consequences of the implementation of a weaning protocol. Intensive Care Med 1996;22(10):1052–6.

[40] Horst HM, Mouro D, Hall-Jenssens RA, et al. Decrease in ventilation time with a standardized weaning process. Arch Surg 1998;133(5):483–8.

[41] Scheinhorn DJ, Chao DC, Stearn-Hassenpflug M, et al. Outcomes in post-ICU mechanical ventilation: a therapist-implemented weaning protocol. Chest 2001;119(1):236–42.

[42] Vitacca M, Vianello A, Colombo D, et al. Comparison of two methods for weaning patients with chronic obstructive pulmonary disease requiring mechanical ventilation for more than 15 days. Am J Respir Crit Care Med 2001;164(2):225–30.

[43] Smyrnios NA, Connolly A, Wilson MM, et al. Effects of a multifaceted, multidisciplinary, hospital-wide quality improvement program on weaning from mechanical ventilation. Crit Care Med 2002; 30(6):1224–30.

[44] Grap MJ, Strickland D, Tormey L, et al. Collaborative practice: development, implementation, and evaluation of a weaning protocol for patients receiving mechanical ventilation. Am J Crit Care 2003; 12(5):454–60.

[45] Dries DJ, McGonigal MD, Malian MS, et al. Protocol-driven ventilator weaning reduces use of mechanical ventilation, rate of early reintubation, and ventilator-associated pneumonia. J Trauma 2004; 56(5):943–51.

[46] Restrepo RD, Fortenberry JD, Spainhour C, et al. Protocol-driven ventilator management in children: comparison to nonprotocol care. J Intensive Care Med 2004;19(5):274–84.

[47] Bumroongkit C, Liwsrisakun C, Deesomchok A, et al. Efficacy of weaning protocol in medical intensive care unit of tertiary care center. J Med Assoc Thai 2005;88(1):52–7.

[48] Tonnelier JM, Prat G, Le Gal G, et al. Impact of a nurses' protocol-directed weaning procedure on outcomes in patients undergoing mechanical ventilation for longer than 48 hours: a prospective cohort study with a matched historical control group. Crit Care 2005;9(2):R83–9.

[49] Aboutanos SZ, Duane TM, Malhotra AK, et al. Prospective evaluation of an extubation protocol in a trauma intensive care unit population. Am Surg 2006;72(5):393–6.

[50] Blackwood B, Wilson-Barnett J, Patterson CC, et al. An evaluation of protocolised weaning on the duration of mechanical ventilation. Anaesthesia 2006; 61(11):1079–86.

[51] Strickland JH Jr, Hasson JH. A computer-controlled ventilator weaning system. A clinical trial. Chest 1993;103(4):1220–6.

[52] Lellouche F, Mancebo J, Jolliet P, et al. A multicenter randomized trial of computer-driven protocolized weaning from mechanical ventilation. Am J Respir Crit Care Med 2006;174(8):894–900.

[53] Kollef MH, Levy NT, Ahrens TS, et al. The use of continuous IV sedation is associated with prolongation of mechanical ventilation. Chest 1998;114(2):541–8.

[54] Brook AD, Ahrens TS, Schaiff R, et al. Effect of a nursing-implemented sedation protocol on the duration of mechanical ventilation. Crit Care Med 1999;27(12):2609–15.

[55] Kress JP, Pohlman AS, O'Connor MF, et al. Daily interruption of sedative infusions in critically ill patients undergoing mechanical ventilation. N Engl J Med 2000;342(20):1471–7.

[56] Djunaedi H, Cardinal P, Greffe-Laliberte G, et al. Does a ventilatory management protocol improve the care of ventilated patients? Respir Care 1997; 42(6):604–10.

ELSEVIER
SAUNDERS

Clin Chest Med 29 (2008) 253–263

CLINICS
IN CHEST
MEDICINE

Controversies in Mechanical Ventilation: When Should a Tracheotomy Be Placed?

Christopher King, MD[a], Lisa K. Moores, MD[b],*

[a]Pulmonary/Critical Care Medicine, Walter Reed Army Medical Center,
3831 Rodman Street Apartment F30, Washington, DC 20016, USA
[b]The Uniformed Services University of the Health Sciences, 4310 Jones Bridge Road, Bethesda, MD 20814, USA

The incidence of disease requiring mechanical ventilation is increasing [1]. Anywhere from 5% to 13% of mechanically ventilated patients will go on to require prolonged support [2]. With such a large and increasing population of mechanically ventilated patients, critical care physicians will frequently face the dilemma of whether to perform tracheotomy. The decision is a complex one, requiring a detailed understanding of the risks and benefits of both tracheotomy and prolonged translaryngeal intubation (TLI). It must also be individualized, taking into consideration the patient's preferences and expected clinical course. This article reviews the medical literature regarding the benefits and risks of tracheotomy as compared with TLI. The authors then discuss current data regarding the optimal timing for the procedure, and propose an algorithm that may aid intensivists in clinical decision making.

Indications for tracheotomy

Tracheotomy has been used for airway management since ancient times [3] and remains one of the most commonly performed intensive care unit procedures [4]. The clinical indications for tracheotomy include relief of upper airway obstruction, assistance with removal of secretions, and provision of airway access for prolonged mechanical ventilation. Examples of airway obstruction requiring tracheotomy are severe maxillofacial trauma, foreign bodies in the upper airway, bilateral vocal cord paralysis, larger tumors of the upper aerodigestive tract, congenital anomalies of the upper airway, laryngeal or tracheal injuries preventing oral or nasal intubation, and swelling of the tongue, pharnynx, larynx, or trachea [3]. While the decision to perform tracheotomy in upper airway obstruction is simple, deciding on the need for and timing of tracheotomy for prolonged mechanical ventilation is complex. It requires a thorough understanding of the possible benefits and complications of placement.

Benefits of tracheotomy

Patient comfort

Though patient comfort is often cited as an advantage of tracheotomy, there are limited data to support this. Astrachan and colleagues [5] surveyed 60 critical care nurses on their attitudes regarding tracheotomy and prolonged TLI. Of those polled, 90% felt that patient comfort was enhanced with tracheotomy and 75% thought patients with tracheotomies fared better psychologically. To the authors' knowledge, no studies have directly surveyed patients undergoing tracheotomy.

A decrease in sedation requirements with tracheotomy is often cited as evidence of improvement in comfort, although the literature supporting this theory is contradictory. Nieszkowska and colleagues [6] performed an observational study in 72 patients undergoing tracheotomy. Sedation

The opinions or assertions contained herein are the private views of the authors and are not to be construed as official or as the views of the Department of the Army or the Department of Defense.

* Corresponding author.
E-mail address: lmoores@usuhs.mil (L.K. Moores).

0272-5231/08/$ - see front matter. Published by Elsevier Inc.
doi:10.1016/j.ccm.2008.01.002

chestmed.theclinics.com

level assessed by Riker's score and the amount of oral and intravenous sedation required in the week before and after tracheotomy were compared. They found a decreased requirement for sedatives and decreased time spent heavily sedated, with no increase in agitation. Because of the study design, it is difficult to tell whether the decreased sedation requirements were attributable to tracheotomy versus clinical improvement. A retrospective study by Veelo and colleagues [7] of 117 patients undergoing tracheotomy compared sedative needs in the week before and after tracheotomy. While a sharp decline in sedation requirements was observed in the days leading up to the procedure, no reduction was observed after tracheotomy. The lack of definitive data for patient comfort and sedation requirements makes it difficult to draw firm conclusions.

Retrospective interviews of patients who underwent TLI revealed that nearly half experienced anxiety or fear while intubated. Inability to communicate was found to be the primary reason for these emotions [8–10]. Tracheotomy affords patients an opportunity for articulated speech. This may reduce anxiety, enhance sense of control and well being, and improve the effectiveness of physician and nursing care. Another advantage of tracheotomy is the potential for oral nutrition. Although swallowing and glottic barrier function may be compromised, resulting in increased risk of aspiration, with the appropriate precautions a tracheotomy does not prevent oral nutrition [11,12]. The ability to take oral nutrition may contribute to improved sense of well being and comfort.

Secure airway

Tracheotomy provides a more secure airway than TLI. Unplanned extubation during TLI has been extensively reported, with rates ranging from 3% to 14% [13–22]. In general, approximately half of patients will require reintubation, with the majority occurring in the first hour. Reintubation is associated with hemodynamic and cardiopulmonary complications in 31% to 72% of patients [16,23]. Additionally, accidental extubation with subsequent reintubation may increase the incidence of nosocomial pneumonia [17,24].

Rates of accidental airway loss in tracheotomy are not as well reported. In the largest series, Goldenberg and colleagues [25] retrospectively studied 1,130 patients undergoing tracheotomy over a 10-year period. They found only four cases of tube obstruction or decannulation (0.35%);

however, all four patients died from this complication. Other series cite event rates of 0% to 7% [26]. Overall, it seems tracheotomy provides a more secure airway than TLI. Tracheotomy also affords greater patient mobility, allowing patients to get out of bed. This may facilitate physical therapy, reduce the likelihood of skin breakdown, enhance patient comfort, and improve the ability to clear airway secretions. This mobility may also allow for transition to lower levels of care or long-term acute care or weaning facilities.

Ventilator associated pneumonia

Ventilator-associated pneumonia (VAP) increases mortality, the length of hospitalization [27] and the duration of mechanical ventilation (MV) [28]. Thus, a thorough understanding of the relationship between tracheotomy and VAP is important to assess the relative benefit of the procedure. Several prospective cohort studies have reported tracheotomy as an independent risk factor for nosocomial pneumonia [27–32]. The majority of these studies fail to establish the timing of tracheotomy in relation to pneumonia; therefore, the higher VAP rate may simply reflect the higher likelihood of prolonged mechanical ventilation in these patients. Only the article by Ibrahim and colleagues [27] specifies timing by noting that tracheotomy was performed before the onset of nosocomial pneumonia in all patients. The study still fails to control for overall duration of MV. Based on this data, it is difficult to ascertain whether tracheotomy is a risk factor for VAP or a marker for longer duration of mechanical ventilation.

Only two studies have tried to control for duration of MV while comparing nosocomial pneumonia rates in patients with prolonged TLI and tracheotomy. Bouderka and colleagues [33] performed a prospective, randomized study in 62 subjecs with severe head injury. Thirty-one subjects undergoing tracheotomy on hospital day five were compared with 31 subjects treated with prolonged TLI. They found no difference in rates of pneumonia between the two groups. Nseir and colleagues [34] performed a retrospective case-control study matching 177 subjects with tracheotomy with 177 control subjects treated with prolonged TLI. They found a statistically significant reduction in VAP episodes per 1,000 mechanical-ventilator days ($P = .009$). In multivariate analysis, tracheotomy was independently associated with a decreased risk for VAP.

Does the timing of the procedure affect the rate of pneumonia? Numerous studies have examined nosocomial pneumonia rates in early versus late tracheotomy [35–46]. The literature on this topic is difficult to interpret because of conflicting results and varying definitions of "early tracheotomy." Two meta-analyses have been performed in attempts to reconcile the disparate data [47,48], with both concluding that early tracheotomy had no influence on rates of nosocomial pneumonia.

Still, with the exception of the article by Rodriguez and colleagues [43], the studies favoring early tracheotomy report lower rates of pneumonia. Differences in the definition of nosocomial pneumonia or in the prophylactic measures taken at individual facilities make comparisons by meta-analysis difficult. A well-designed randomized trial may still prove early tracheotomy superior in reducing rates of nosocomial pneumonia. However, current evidence does not allow the authors to draw definitive conclusions other than stating that early tracheotomy is unlikely to result in an increase in risk. Larger randomized, controlled trials comparing tracheotomy to prolonged TLI are needed to answer this question.

Weaning from mechanical ventilation

The effect that tracheotomy has on weaning from mechanical ventilation is often debated. Proposed reasons for facilitated weaning include: (1) reduced dead space, (2) decreased airway resistance and work of breathing, (3) improved removal of secretions, (4) decreased need for sedation, (5) improved patient comfort, and (6) decreased rates of VAP [49]. The issues of VAP, patient comfort, and sedation have been covered in detail above.

Several groups have addressed the difference in dead space between tracheostomy and endotracheal tubes (ETTs). Davis and colleagues [50] compared the dead space of standard ETTs with tracheostomy tubes and found that the differences were less than 20 mL. Mohr and colleagues [51] assessed the clinical significance of these small differences in dead space by calculating dead space (V_d/V_t) via capnography in 45 patients 24 hours before and after tracheotomy. They found no significant difference between the pre- and posttracheotomy V_d/V_t (50.73 plus or minus 10.5 versus 51.88 plus or minus 11.4, $P = .31$). Given the above, it seems unlikely that changes in dead space play a significant role in facilitating weaning.

Work of breathing

Reduction in tube resistance leading to a decreased work of breathing is a more plausible reason for weaning benefits after tracheotomy. Increased resistance in a tube will be seen with decreases in diameter, increases in length, luminal irregularities, higher gas flow rates, and curves in the tube [49]. Davis and Porembka [52] studied work of breathing in ETTs and tracheostomy tubes of various sizes. Imposed work of breathing in a tracheostomy tube was lower than in an ETT of equivalent inner diameter. Four studies have compared work of breathing before and after tracheotomy [50,53–56]. Lin and colleagues [55] found no change in work of breathing, although a decrease in peak inspiratory pressure was noted. The other studies all demonstrated a significant decrease in work of breathing. The differences in work of breathing and tube resistance are small in these studies, but with increased minute ventilation the effects will be magnified. Still, this may not translate to improvements in clinical outcomes, such as time spent weaning from mechanical ventilation.

Weaning trials are often limited by methodologic flaws. Providers cannot be blinded to intervention, and physicians may be more willing to discontinue ventilatory support in patients with a tracheotomy. Additionally, variations in weaning protocols, populations studied, timing of tracheotomy, and the definition of "weaning" make direct comparison between studies difficult.

Though numerous trials have examined the effects of tracheotomy on weaning times, the authors will focus only on those that are randomized and controlled (RCTs). Five RCTs have compared early tracheotomy to prolonged TLI or late tracheotomy using duration of mechanical ventilation as the outcomes measure [33,36,43–45]. Three of the five [33,43,44] found a significant reduction in ventilatory days in the early tracheotomy groups. Griffiths and colleagues [48] performed a meta-analysis with four of the five studies (Bouderka and colleagues [33] was not published yet) and found that early tracheotomy significantly reduced the duration of mechanical ventilation, with a weighted mean difference of −8.5 days. The results of this analysis are at odds with those of a previous systematic review by Maziak and colleagues [57]. However, two of the five articles reviewed by Maziak are retrospective in nature [37,41]. A third article cited doesn't actually report a mean duration of mechanical ventilation [39]. Given the available data, tracheotomy, particularly when performed early, appears to reduce the duration of mechanical ventilation. The mechanisms behind this reduction and the appropriate patient population required to maximize this benefit are unclear.

Risks of tracheotomy

Despite being a commonly performed procedure, tracheotomy is not risk free. Clinicians must consider the risk of immediate and long-term complications, as well as the time and expense of the procedure. This section briefly discusses commonly performed techniques and the contraindications to tracheotomy. The authors will then review the reported rates of early and late complications associated with the procedure.

Techniques

In the early 1900s, Chevalier Jackson popularized an open surgical approach to tracheotomy [58]. Open surgical techniques were the mainstay throughout the twentieth century, but over the last 15 years percutaneous procedures have become increasingly popular. A recent meta-analysis [58] comparing fifteen RCTs revealed a trend toward reduced complications with the percutaneous approach. The investigators also found percutaneous tracheotomies were more cost-effective (with an average savings of $456 USD) and of shorter case length (average 4.6 minutes). Recent guidelines released by the Belgian Society of Pneumology and the Belgian Association for Cardiothoracic Surgery recommend percutaneous dilational tracheotomy as the procedure of choice for elective tracheotomy in critically ill adult patients [59].

The time, inconvenience, and risk for complications with transfer to an operating room (OR) are often cited as a disadvantage of performing tracheotomy. Studies have demonstrated that both percutaneous and open tracheotomies can safely be performed at the bedside [26,60–65]. Selected location is based on the standard practice and comfort level of the practitioners performing the procedure, but bedside placement is acceptable and may be preferable to transferring the patient to the OR.

Contraindications

There are few absolute contraindications to tracheotomy. They include patient refusal, skin infection at the operative site, and prior neck surgery that obscures neck anatomy [59]. Several other special situations deserve comment, but none present an absolute contraindication. Morbid obesity may increase complication rates in both open and percutaneous tracheotomy [66,67], but with caution both can be safely performed [68,69]. Patients with thrombocytopenia can undergo tracheotomy with platelet transfusion before the procedure [59]. Heparin products should temporarily be discontinued in patients requiring anticoagulation [59].

Complications

Complications are reported in 5% to 40% of tracheotomies [25]. In their retrospective analysis of 1,130 subjects, Goldenberg and colleagues [25] found a major complication rate of 4.3% with 0.7% mortality. Reported events were divided into three specific time periods. Perioperative complications included bleeding, cardiopulmonary arrest, hypoxia because of airway loss, damage to adjacent anatomic structures (such as the recurrent laryngeal nerve or the esophagus), and rare intraoperative fires caused by electrocautery [25]. Early postoperative complications included bleeding, pneumothorax or pneumomediastinum, tube decannulation or obstruction, and wound infection. Bleeding is the most common occurrence among these, with the others rarely reported. It is largely preventable with careful surgical technique [70]. In the retrospective series by Goldenberg and colleagues, hemorrhage was the most common early complication with a rate of 0.8% [25], although other series report rates between 1% and 37% [26].

Pneumothorax, subcutaneous emphysema, or pneumomediastinum can occur secondary to dissection of air along soft-tissue planes, direct damage to the pleura, or rupture of a bleb [70]. Goldenberg reported a rate of 0.34% for pneumothorax and subcutaneous emphysema, with two deaths resulting from tension pneumothorax [25]. Tube decannulation or obstruction can be a devastating complication in the early postoperative period before a mature stoma is formed. Goldenberg reported a rate of only 0.35% for this complication, with 100% mortality [25]. Higgins and Punthakee performed a meta-analysis comparing complications between open and percutaneous tracheotomy. In their study, 10 trials reported on decannulation or obstruction. When data from these studies are pooled, there were

29 events of decannulation or obstruction in 742 subjects, a rate of 3.9% [58].

Wound infection is another common early complication in tracheotomy. Goldenberg and colleagues [25] reported a low infection rate of 0.44%, all of which resolved with treatment. Higgins and Punthakee [58] found 13 trials reporting on wound infection or stomatitis after tracheotomy. Pooled event rates from these studies reveal 73 infections in 850 subjects, a rate of 8.6%. The authors suspect the pooled data from the RCTs given above more closely reflects actual event rates, as complications were being actively sought, rather than assessed retrospectively by chart review.

Tracheal stenosis is a commonly cited late complication of both TLI and tracheotomy. Pressure exerted by the tube and its cuff are thought to impair mucosal capillary perfusion, eventually resulting in mucosal ulceration. The ulcerations will heal by fibrosis and result in progressive stenosis [71]. Whited [72] found that longer duration of intubation was associated with increased rates of stenosis, with a 2% incidence with less than 6 days, 5% with 6 to 10 days, and 12% with greater than 10 days of intubation. Rates of symptomatic tracheal stenosis following tracheotomy are relatively low, with estimates of 1% to 12% [59,73]. Twenty-one cases were reported in 1,130 patients (1.85%) in the retrospective series by Goldenberg and colleagues [25]. TLI can also result in stenosis, but relative rates following TLI and tracheotomy are not known.

Tracheo-innominate artery fistula is a rare (less than 0.07%) but a devastating late complication of tracheotomy, with a survival rate of only 25%. Fistulas occur when the cannula erodes through the innominate artery [59]. Tracheo-esophageal fistula is also rare, with an estimated incidence of less than 1%. It is an iatrogenic injury resulting from compromise of the posterior tracheal wall during placement. Repair generally requires thoracic surgery, although stenting is an option in some patients [73]. Tracheo-cutaneous fistulas and dysphagia are also late complications of tracheotomy.

Impact on outcome in critically ill patients

The effect of tracheotomy on intensive care unit (ICU), hospital, and overall outcomes is also controversial. To date, there is only one prospective, RCT comparing early versus late tracheotomy [43], and none comparing tracheotomy versus persistent TLI in the general ICU population. A more recent RCT restricted to severe head injured patients found no difference in outcome between tracheotomy and TLI patients [33].

The remainder of the data on outcomes are retrospective and involve heterogeneous patient populations, yielding conflicting results. Frutos-Vivar and colleagues [74] performed an observational cohort study of over 5,000 patients, from 361 ICUs in 12 countries, who were mechanically ventilated longer than 12 hours. The investigators sought to determine the prevalence and timing of tracheotomy, the clinical conditions associated with its placement, and outcomes as measured by ICU and hospital length of stay (LOS) and mortality. Patients with a tracheotomy had longer ICU (21 days versus 7 days) and hospital (36 days versus 15 days) LOS. Mortality in the ICU was lower in patients who received a tracheotomy (20% versus 32%). Adjusting for other variables, tracheotomy was independently related to survival in the ICU (odds ratio 2.22; 95% confidence index 1.72–2.86). Hospital mortality was not different between the groups. The study's observational design precludes strong conclusions.

Two publications in the past year sought to clarify this issue. The first was a retrospective review that attempted to limit confounding by using a nested case-control design, enrolling subjects admitted during the same time period [75]. The investigators found tracheotomy was associated with lower ICU and hospital mortality rates, even after adjusting for physiologic variables on admission and on day three. The study was limited by its retrospective design and potential for considerable selection bias. In addition, the investigators did not collect information about weaning failure, reintubation rates, or decisions to withhold or withdraw life-sustaining treatments.

The second, most recent study was prospective and observational, enrolling unselected subjects requiring MV for greater than or equal to 48 hours in 12 French ICUs over a 7-year period [76]. The investigators matched each tracheotomy subject with two controls, each selected according to the likelihood of undergoing the procedure. They found tracheotomy did not improve ICU mortality and was associated with more days of MV and longer ICU LOS. Still, the methods used for matching have limitations, and larger, well-designed studies are needed before firm conclusions can be drawn. In addition, future studies might also examine after ICU quality of life as another important outcome in these patients.

Three systematic reviews have attempted to address the issue of tracheotomy timing and ultimate outcomes. In his 1998 review, Maziak [57] performed a systematic review of three randomized and two retrospective studies. Because of flaws in the randomization techniques and varying definitions of "early," no conclusions could be made. In 2005, Griffiths and colleagues [48] published an updated systematic review and meta-analysis. The investigators identified five prospective randomized trials that addressed timing: two included in the Maziak review, and three more recently published trials. There was significant heterogeneity among all trials, with varying inclusion and exclusion criteria and definitions of what constituted early or late tracheotomy. Populations varied across studies (head injury, trauma, burn, medical, and general surgical patients were included). Using a random effects model, the investigators concluded that early tracheotomy was associated with shorter duration of mechanical ventilation and ICU days, but had no effect on overall mortality [48].

A third review focused exclusively on the trauma population. Dunham and Ransom [47] identified seven retrospective comparisons of early versus late tracheotomy, five randomized trials of early tracheotomy versus no tracheotomy, and one randomized trial of early versus late tracheotomy. Although outcome data was extracted and summarized from all trials, only RCTs were combined using meta-analytic techniques. The investigators found no difference in mortality with early tracheotomy. Of note, because of significant heterogeneity, the RCT comparing early versus late tracheotomy was excluded from the final analysis. Results of this trial relate solely to outcomes in trauma patients and fail to answer the question of optimal timing. Limitations in the existing evidence base preclude definitive conclusions regarding the effect of timing on ultimate outcomes. Currently, there are three large scale, appropriately powered RCTs ongoing. When completed, they may provide the evidence needed for informed decision making [77–79].

Putting it all together

Because of gaps in the literature, tracheotomy practice varies considerably. Nathens and colleagues [80] examined procedure rates in over 17,000 trauma patients from approximately 100 centers across the United States entered into the National Trauma Databank from 2001 to 2003. They found the rate of tracheotomy varied from 0 to 59 per 100 hospital admissions. Although several patient characteristics were predictive of the procedure, they explained only 14% of the variance across centers. Eighty percent of the variance could not be explained by either patient or institutional characteristics, suggesting a true lack of adequate higher level evidence to guide practice. The Belgian Association of Cardiothoracic Surgery recently published a clinical review and evidence-based guidelines [59], but the authors were unable to make any strong, high level recommendations about indications or timing of tracheotomy.

In many ways we still must follow Dr. Heffner, who recommended an "anticipatory" approach to tracheotomy 15 years ago [81]. Performance of the procedure should be done after careful review of the risks and benefits—individualized to the patient. A general approach considers tracheotomy after the patient has undergone some period of stabilization. Patients likely to be liberated from the ventilator within 7 to 10 days continue with an endotracheal tube in place. In contrast, those requiring a longer duration could be offered tracheotomy. When duration cannot be predicted, patients can be re-evaluated on a daily basis. This anticipatory approach assumes that clinicians can accurately predict the duration of mechanical ventilation early in the patient's clinical course.

Predicting the duration of mechanical ventilation

In patients with traumatic brain injury, a Glasgow Coma Scale (GCS) score of less than or equal to 6 on day four of the ICU course indicates prolonged ventilatory support will be needed [82,83]. Prediction is less precise in patients with acute neuromuscular disease, such as Guillain-Barré syndrome. Those who are elderly, display signs of autonomic dysfunction, or have pre-existing lung disease often require prolonged MV and should be considered for early tracheotomy [84,85].

Seneff and colleagues [86] attempted to develop a prediction equation in a large population of mixed ICU patients. Using APACHE III (acute physiology, age, and chronic health evaluation) data from almost 6,000 ICU patients at 40 United States hospitals, the investigators performed multivariate regression analysis to determine if particular patient or disease characteristics on day one could be used to determine the duration of mechanical ventilation. They found that admitting diagnosis and degree of physiologic derangement measured by the Acute Physiology Score could accurately predict duration of mechanical ventilation in groups of ICU patients. Although this might prove useful for comparing ventilator practices between different ICUs, it is not useful for predicting the duration of mechanical ventilation in individual patients.

Troche and Moine [87] used data from 195 consecutive patients admitted to their surgical ICU over a 12-month period to determine if clinical or physiologic parameters on admission or at the time of intubation could be used to predict the need for mechanical ventilation for more than 14 days. Only emergency intubation and a Lung Injury Score (LIS) greater than or equal to

1 independently predicted a duration of more than 14 days. In a separate validation phase of the study in 128 consecutive patients who required emergent intubation, the utility of the LIS less than 1 was in its negative predictive value (91%), rather than the positive predictive value (0.24) [87]. Study patients had a low overall rate of prolonged MV and were from a single surgical ICU, but in patients with an LIS less than 1, early tracheotomy should not be considered.

An earlier retrospective study reported on 91 subjects admitted to the surgical ICU at a level 1 trauma center over a 3-month period [88]. Thirty percent of the cohort required MV for longer than 14 days. Clinical and physiologic variables in these subjects on day two were compared with the patients who required MV for less than 14 days. The investigators found that a day two GCS of less than or equal to 9 or a day two

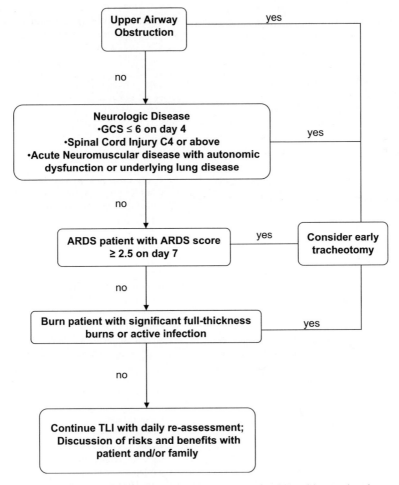

Fig. 1. A suggested algorithm using Heffner's "Anticipatory Approach" and integrating the current data.

alveolar-arterial oxygen gradient greater than or equal to 175 mm HG in subjects without preexisting chronic obstructive lung disease had a sensitivity of 91% and a specificity of 96% for requirement of ventilatory support for 14 days or more. To the authors' knowledge, this approach has not been prospectively validated.

Heffner and Zamora [89] developed an Acute Respiratory Distress Syndrome (ARDS) Predictive Score, then tested prospectively for accuracy in predicting an uncomplicated ARDS course (defined as MV requirement of less than 14 days) [90]. The score was calculated on days four and seven in 50 patients with ARDS in the critical care units of a large Academic Medical Center over a 4-year period. An ARDS Score of greater than or equal to 2.5 accurately identified patients at risk of prolonged intubation.

Finally, Sellers and colleagues [91] reviewed the charts of 110 burn patients over a 4-year period who required MV for at least 3 days. They used logistic regression to develop an equation to predict those patients that would require more than 14 days of MV. Using 29 patients admitted the following year as a prospective validation cohort, the equation was found to have 100% positive predictive value.

In summary, tools have been developed that may help us predict the duration of MV in select populations of patients, but more robust external validation is needed. In addition, more research should be done in the other populations who often require prolonged MV, such as patients with sepsis and chronic obstructive lung disease.

A suggested algorithm

Using Heffner's "Anticipatory Approach" and integrating the current data, the authors propose the approach presented in Fig. 1.

References

[1] Carson SS, Cox CE, Holmes GM, et al. The changing epidemiology of mechanical ventilation: a population-based study. J Intensive Care Med 2006;21(3):173–82.
[2] Nevins ML, Epstein SK. Weaning from prolonged mechanical ventilation. Clin Chest Med 2001;22(1): 13–33.
[3] Wenig BL, Applebaum EL. Indications for and techniques of tracheotomy. Clin Chest Med 1991; 12(3):545–53.
[4] Durbin CG Jr. Indications for and timing of tracheostomy. Respir Care 2005;50(4):483–7.
[5] Astrachan DI, Kirchner JC, Goodwin WJ Jr. Prolonged intubation vs. tracheotomy: complications, practical and psychological considerations. Laryngoscope 1988;98(11):1165–9.
[6] Nieszkowska A, Combes A, Luyt CE, et al. Impact of tracheotomy on sedative administration, sedation level, and comfort of mechanically ventilated intensive care unit patients. Crit Care Med 2005; 33(11):2527–33.
[7] Veelo DP, Dongelmans DA, Binnekade JM, et al. Tracheotomy does not affect reducing sedation requirements of patients in intensive care—a retrospective study. Crit Care 2006;10(4):R99.
[8] Bergbom-Engberg I, Haljamae H. Assessment of patients' experience of discomforts during respirator therapy. Crit Care Med 1989;17(10):1068–72.
[9] Leder SB. Importance of verbal communication for the ventilator-dependent patient. Chest 1990;98(4): 792–3.
[10] Pochard F, Lanore JJ, Bellivier F, et al. Subjective psychological status of severely ill patients discharged from mechanical ventilation. Clin Intensive Care 1995;6(2):57–61.
[11] Godwin JE, Heffner JE. Special critical care considerations in tracheostomy management. Clin Chest Med 1991;12(3):573–83.
[12] Murray KA, Brzozowski LA. Swallowing in patients with tracheotomies. AACN Clin Issues 1998;9(3): 416–26 [quiz 456–8].
[13] Betbese AJ, Perez M, Bak E, et al. A prospective study of unplanned endotracheal extubation in intensive care unit patients. Crit Care Med 1998; 26(7):1180–6.
[14] Boulain T. Unplanned extubations in the adult intensive care unit: a prospective multicenter study. Association des Reanimateurs du Centre-Ouest. Am J Respir Crit Care Med 1998;157(4 Pt 1):1131–7.
[15] Chevron V, Menard JF, Richard JC, et al. Unplanned extubation: risk factors of development and predictive criteria for reintubation. Crit Care Med 1998;26(6):1049–53.
[16] Coppolo DP, May JJ. Self-extubations. A 12-month experience. Chest 1990;98(1):165–9.
[17] de Lassence A, Alberti C, Azoulay E, et al. Impact of unplanned extubation and reintubation after weaning on nosocomial pneumonia risk in the intensive care unit: a prospective multicenter study. Anesthesiology 2002;97(1):148–56.
[18] Esteban A, Anzueto A, Frutos F, et al. Characteristics and outcomes in adult patients receiving mechanical ventilation: a 28-day international study. JAMA 2002;287(3):345–55.
[19] Listello D, Sessler CN. Unplanned extubation. Clinical predictors for reintubation. Chest 1994; 105(5):1496–503.
[20] Razek T, Gracias V, Sullivan D, et al. Assessing the need for reintubation: a prospective evaluation of unplanned endotracheal extubation. J Trauma 2000;48(3):466–9.

[21] Tindol GA Jr, DiBenedetto RJ, Kosciuk L. Unplanned extubations. Chest 1994;105(6):1804–7.

[22] Vassal T, Anh NG, Gabillet JM, et al. Prospective evaluation of self-extubations in a medical intensive care unit. Intensive Care Med 1993;19(6):340–2.

[23] Mort TC. Unplanned tracheal extubation outside the operating room: a quality improvement audit of hemodynamic and tracheal airway complications associated with emergency tracheal reintubation. Anesth Analg 1998;86(6):1171–6.

[24] Torres A, Gatell JM, Aznar E, et al. Re-intubation increases the risk of nosocomial pneumonia in patients needing mechanical ventilation. Am J Respir Crit Care Med 1995;152(1):137–41.

[25] Goldenberg D, Ari EG, Golz A, et al. Tracheotomy complications: a retrospective study of 1130 cases. Otolaryngol Head Neck Surg 2000;123(4):495–500.

[26] Goldstein SI, Breda SD, Schneider KL. Surgical complications of bedside tracheotomy in an otolaryngology residency program. Laryngoscope 1987;97(12):1407–9.

[27] Ibrahim EH, Tracy L, Hill C, et al. The occurrence of ventilator-associated pneumonia in a community hospital: risk factors and clinical outcomes. Chest 2001;120(2):555–61.

[28] Apostolopoulou E, Bakakos P, Katostaras T, et al. Incidence and risk factors for ventilator-associated pneumonia in 4 multidisciplinary intensive care units in Athens, Greece. Respir Care 2003;48:681–8.

[29] Alp E, Guven M, Yildiz O, et al. Incidence, risk factors and mortality of nosocomial pneumonia in intensive care units: a prospective study. Ann Clin Microbiol Antimicrob 2004;3:17.

[30] Carrilho CM, Grion CM, Bonametti AM, et al. Multivariate analysis of the factors associated with the risk of pneumonia in intensive care units. Braz J Infect Dis 2007;11(3):339–44.

[31] Erbay H, Yalcin AN, Serin S, et al. Nosocomial infections in intensive care unit in a Turkish university hospital: a 2-year survey. Intensive Care Med 2003;29(9):1482–8.

[32] Tejada Artigas A, Bello Dronda S, Chacon Valles E, et al. Risk factors for nosocomial pneumonia in critically ill trauma patients. Crit Care Med 2001; 29(2):304–9.

[33] Bouderka MA, Fakhir B, Bouaggad A, et al. Early tracheostomy versus prolonged endotracheal intubation in severe head injury. J Trauma 2004; 57(2):251–4.

[34] Nseir S, Di Pompeo C, Jozefowicz E, et al. Relationship between tracheotomy and ventilator-associated pneumonia: a case control study. Eur Respir J 2007; 30(2):314–20.

[35] Armstrong PA, McCarthy MC, Peoples JB. Reduced use of resources by early tracheostomy in ventilator-dependent patients with blunt trauma. Surgery 1998;124(4):763–6 [discussion: 766–7].

[36] Barquist ES, Amortegui J, Hallal A, et al. Tracheostomy in ventilator dependent trauma patients: a prospective, randomized intention-to-treat study. J Trauma 2006;60(1):91–7.

[37] Blot F, Guiguet M, Antonn S, et al. Early tracheotomy in neutropenic, mechanically ventilated patients: rational and results of pilot study. Support Care Cancer 1995;3:291–6.

[38] Brook AD, Sherman G, Malen J, et al. Early versus late tracheostomy in patients who require prolonged mechanical ventilation. Am J Crit Care 2000;9(5): 352–9.

[39] Dunham CM, LaMonica C. Prolonged tracheal intubation in the trauma patient. J Trauma 1984; 24(2):120–4.

[40] Kluger Y, Paul DB, Lucke J, et al. Early tracheostomy in trauma patients. Eur J Emerg Med 1996; 3(2):95–101.

[41] Lesnik I, Rappaport W, Fulginiti J, et al. The role of early tracheostomy in blunt, multiple organ trauma. Am Surg 1992;58(6):346–9.

[42] Moller MG, Slaikeu JD, Bonelli P, et al. Early tracheostomy versus late tracheostomy in the surgical intensive care unit. Am J Surg 2005;189(3): 293–6.

[43] Rodriguez JL, Steinberg SM, Luchetti FA, et al. Early tracheostomy for primary airway management in the surgical critical care setting. Surgery 1990;108(4):655–9.

[44] Rumbak MJ, Newton M, Truncale T, et al. A prospective, randomized, study comparing early percutaneous dilational tracheotomy to prolonged translaryngeal intubation (delayed tracheotomy) in critically ill medical patients. Crit Care Med 2004; 32(8):1689–94.

[45] Saffle JR, Morris SE, Edelman L. Early tracheostomy does not improve outcome in burn patients. J Burn Care Rehabil 2002;23(6):431–8.

[46] Sugerman HJ, Wolfe L, Pasquale MD, et al. Multicenter, randomized, prospective trial of early tracheostomy. J Trauma 1997;43(5):741–7.

[47] Dunham CM, Ransom KJ. Assessment of early tracheostomy in trauma patients: a systematic review and meta-analysis. Am Surg 2006;72(3):276–81.

[48] Griffiths J, Barber VS, Morgan L, et al. Systematic review and meta-analysis of studies of the timing of tracheostomy in adult patients undergoing artificial ventilation. BMJ 2005;330(7502):1243.

[49] Pierson DJ. Tracheostomy and weaning. Respir Care 2005;50(4):526–33.

[50] Davis K Jr, Campbell RS, Johannigman JA, et al. Changes in respiratory mechanics after tracheostomy. Arch Surg 1999;134(1):59–62.

[51] Mohr AM, Rutherford EJ, Cairns BA, et al. The role of dead space ventilation in predicting outcome of successful weaning from mechanical ventilation. J Trauma 2001;51(5):843–8.

[52] Davis K Jr, Branson RD, Porembka D. A comparison of the imposed work of breathing with endotracheal and tracheostomy tubes in a lung model. Respir Care 1994;39(6):611–6.

[53] Amygdalou A, Dimopoulos G, Moukas M, et al. Immediate post-operative effects of tracheotomy on respiratory function during mechanical ventilation. Crit Care 2004;8(4):R243–7.

[54] Diehl JL, El Atrous S, Touchard D, et al. Changes in the work of breathing induced by tracheotomy in ventilator-dependent patients. Am J Respir Crit Care Med 1999;159(2):383–8.

[55] Lin MC, Huang CC, Yang CT, et al. Pulmonary mechanics in patients with prolonged mechanical ventilation requiring tracheostomy. Anaesth Intensive Care 1999;27(6):581–5.

[56] Moscovici da Cruz V, Demarzo SE, Sobrinho JB, et al. Effects of tracheotomy on respiratory mechanics in spontaneously breathing patients. Eur Respir J 2002;20(1):112–7.

[57] Maziak DE, Meade MO, Todd TR. The timing of tracheotomy: a systematic review. Chest 1998; 114(2):605–9.

[58] Higgins KM, Punthakee X. Meta-analysis comparison of open versus percutaneous tracheostomy. Laryngoscope 2007;117(3):447–54.

[59] De Leyn P, Bedert L, Delcroix M, et al. Tracheotomy: clinical review and guidelines. Eur J Cardiothorac Surg 2007;32(3):412–21.

[60] Cobean R, Beals M, Moss C, et al. Percutaneous dilatational tracheostomy. A safe, cost-effective bedside procedure. Arch Surg 1996;131(3):265–71.

[61] Pogue MD, Pecaro BC. Safety and efficiency of elective tracheostomy performed in the intensive care unit. J Oral Maxillofac Surg 1995;53(8):895–7.

[62] Upadhyay A, Maurer J, Turner J, et al. Elective bedside tracheostomy in the intensive care unit. J Am Coll Surg 1996;183(1):51–5.

[63] Wang SJ, Sercarz JA, Blackwell KE, et al. Open bedside tracheotomy in the intensive care unit. Laryngoscope 1999;109(6):891–3.

[64] Wease GL, Frikker M, Villalba M, et al. Bedside tracheostomy in the intensive care unit. Arch Surg 1996;131(5):552–4 [discussion: 554–5].

[65] Winkler WB, Karnik R, Seelmann O, et al. Bedside percutaneous dilational tracheostomy with endoscopic guidance: experience with 71 ICU patients. Intensive Care Med 1994;20(7):476–9.

[66] Byhahn C, Lischke V, Meininger D, et al. Perioperative complications during percutaneous tracheostomy in obese patients. Anaesthesia 2005; 60(1):12–5.

[67] El Solh AA, Jaafar W. A comparative study of the complications of surgical tracheostomy in morbidly obese critically ill patients. Crit Care 2007; 11(1):R3.

[68] Heyrosa MG, Melniczek DM, Rovito P, et al. Percutaneous tracheostomy: a safe procedure in the morbidly obese. J Am Coll Surg 2006;202(4):618–22.

[69] Mansharamani NG, Koziel H, Garland R, et al. Safety of bedside percutaneous dilatational tracheostomy in obese patients in the ICU. Chest 2000; 117(5):1426–9.

[70] Myers EN, Carrau RL. Early complications of tracheotomy. Incidence and management. Clin Chest Med 1991;12(3):589–95.

[71] Sue RD, Susanto I. Long-term complications of artificial airways. Clin Chest Med 2003;24(3): 457–71.

[72] Whited RE. A prospective study of laryngotracheal sequelae in long-term intubation. Laryngoscope 1984;94(3):367–77.

[73] Epstein SK. Late complications of tracheostomy. Respir Care 2005;50(4):542–9.

[74] Frutos-Vivar F, Esteban A, Apezteguia C, et al. Outcome of mechanically ventilated patients who require a tracheostomy. Crit Care Med 2005;33(2): 290–8.

[75] Combes A, Luyt CE, Nieszkowska A, et al. Is tracheostomy associated with better outcomes for patients requiring long-term mechanical ventilation? Crit Care Med 2007;35(3):802–7.

[76] Clec'h C, Alberti C, Vincent F, et al. Tracheostomy does not improve the outcome of patients requiring prolonged mechanical ventilation: a propensity analysis. Crit Care Med 2007;35(1):132–8.

[77] Tracheostomy Management in Critical Care (TracMan). Available at: http://www.controlled-trials.com/mrct/trial/238273/TracMAn. Accessed 31 December, 2007.

[78] Early Percutaneous Tracheostomy for Cardiac Surgery (ETOC). Available at: http://www.clinical trials.gov/ct/show/NCT00347321. Accessed 31 December, 2007.

[79] Early Versus Late Tracheostomy. Available at: http://www.clinicaltrials.gov/ct/show/NCT00262431. Accessed 31 December, 2007.

[80] Nathens AB, Rivara FP, Mack CD, et al. Variations in rates of tracheostomy in the critically ill trauma patient. Crit Care Med 2006;34(12):2919–24.

[81] Heffner JE. Timing of tracheotomy in mechanically ventilated patients. Am Rev Respir Dis 1993;147(3): 768–71.

[82] Koh WY, Lew TW, Chin NM, et al. Tracheostomy in a neuro-intensive care setting: indications and timing. Anaesth Intensive Care 1997;25(4):365–8.

[83] Major KM, Hui T, Wilson MT, et al. Objective indications for early tracheostomy after blunt head trauma. Am J Surg 2003;186(6):615–9 [discussion: 619].

[84] Lawn ND, Wijdicks EF. Tracheostomy in Guillain-Barré syndrome. Muscle Nerve 1999;22(8):1058–62.

[85] Nguyen TN, Badjatia N, Malhotra A, et al. Factors predicting extubation success in patients with Guillain-Barré syndrome. Neurocrit Care 2006; 5(3):230–4.

[86] Seneff MG, Zimmerman JE, Knaus WA, et al. Predicting the duration of mechanical ventilation. The importance of disease and patient characteristics. Chest 1996;110(2):469–79.

[87] Troche G, Moine P. Is the duration of mechanical ventilation predictable? Chest 1997;112(3):745–51.

[88] Johnson SB, Kearney PA, Barker DE. Early criteria predictive of prolonged mechanical ventilation. J Trauma 1992;33(1):95–100.

[89] Heffner JE, Zamora CA. Clinical predictors of prolonged translaryngeal intubation in patients with the adult respiratory distress syndrome. Chest 1990;97(2):447–52 [%R 10.1378/chest.97.2.447].

[90] Heffner JE, Brown LK, Barbieri CA, et al. Prospective validation of an acute respiratory distress syndrome predictive score. Am J Respir Crit Care Med 1995;152(5):1518–26.

[91] Sellers BJ, Davis BL, Larkin PW, et al. Early prediction of prolonged ventilator dependence in thermally injured patients. J Trauma 1997;43(6):899–903.

ELSEVIER
SAUNDERS

Clin Chest Med 29 (2008) 265–275

CLINICS
IN CHEST
MEDICINE

Current Role of High Frequency Oscillatory Ventilation and Airway Pressure Release Ventilation in Acute Lung Injury and Acute Respiratory Distress Syndrome

Chuin Siau, MBBS, MRCP[a,1], Thomas E. Stewart, MD, FRCPC[a,b,c,*]

[a]*Interdepartmental Division of Critical Care Medicine, University of Toronto, 220 Victoria Street, Suite 1807, Toronto, Ontario, Canada M5B 2R6*
[b]*Critical Care Unit, Mount Sinai Hospital, Suite 18-206, 600 University Avenue, Toronto, Ontario, Canada M5G 1X5*
[c]*Critical Care Unit, University Health Network, 190 Elizaberth Street, Toronto, Ontario, Canada M5G 2C4*

Acute lung injury (ALI) and acute respiratory distress syndrome (ARDS) continue to be associated with high morbidity, mortality [1–4], and socioeconomic burden [1,4]. Despite advances in the understanding of the pathophysiology of ALI and ARDS, no effective therapeutic intervention has been identified [5]. As a result, supportive care, of which mechanical ventilation is the cornerstone, is in essence all a clinician can offer. Despite the fact that mechanical ventilation is essential, it has potential deleterious effects that negatively impact on morbidity and mortality. Ventilator induced lung injury (VILI) [6,7] can occur through high inflation pressures and alveolar over-distension (barotrauma and volutrauma), repetitive recruitment and derecruitment (atelectrauma), and oxygen toxicity. Direct physical injuries to the alveoli delivered via mechanical ventilation may also stimulate the release of inflammatory mediators (biotrauma). These inflammatory mediators have been implicated in the exacerbation of local lung damage, and by virtue

of their ability to overflow into the systemic circulation, there is a possible link to the development of multiorgan failure [8,9]. The latter is the primary cause of death in patients with ALI and ARDS [9].

Historically, high tidal volumes (V_Ts) (eg, 12 mL/kg–15 mL/kg) [10] have been used in efforts to attain normal blood gases. Often, this is achieved at the expense of subjecting the lungs to excessive stress and strain. To minimize the risk of VILI, lung protection strategies have been developed and tested with the primary aim of protecting the patient's lungs and a secondary emphasis on normalizing blood gases [11]. Although there have been a number of randomized, controlled studies evaluating various lung protective approaches using conventional ventilators, only a few have found a difference in mortality.

In the first trial of 53 subjects, Amato and colleagues [12] were able to demonstrate a significant 28-day mortality reduction (38% versus 71%, $P < .001$) using a lung protective strategy with high positive end-expiratory pressure (PEEP) and recruitment maneuvers (RM) over a conventional ventilation approach, which emphasized normalization of carbon dioxide levels. Despite the fact that this was the first trial to confirm that approaches to conventional mechanical ventilation can influence outcome, the control arm—which had a very high mortality—may have accounted for the survival difference. Nonetheless,

[1] Mailing address for Chuin Siau as of July 1, 2008: Department of Medicine, Changi General Hospital, 2 Simei Street 3, S(529889), Singapore.
* Corresponding author. Mount Sinai Hospital, Suite 18-206, 600 University Avenue, Toronto, Ontario, Canada M5G 1X5.
E-mail address: tstewart@mtsinai.on.ca (T.E. Stewart).

the intervention arm—which incorporated several aspects of lung protection (pressure and volume limitation, high PEEP, and RMs)—had impressive outcomes that have subsequently been evaluated in varying degrees [13–15]. Another trial that found a mortality difference was by the National Heart, Lung and Blood Institute ARDS Network (ARDSNet) [16]. In this trial, the investigators focused on pressure and volume limitation. Using a protocol (target V_T of 6-mL/kg predicted body weight and keeping plateau pressure less than or equal to 30 cm H_2O), the investigators conducted a randomized, controlled trial on 861 subjects, showing a 9% absolute reduction in mortality (31% versus 39.8%, $P = .007$).

Undoubtedly, lung protective mechanical ventilation using conventional ventilation has become the standard of care. A recent study by Terragni and colleagues [17], however, showed that despite adopting ARDSNet protocol [16], aerated lungs are at risk of tidal hyperinflation in ARDS patients with large dependent, nonaerated compartments. These results suggest that rather than adopting a universal approach to mechanical ventilation, ventilatory strategies should be individualized, attending to the specific needs of patients and their disease process.

What is unknown is the extent to which unconventional approaches may be able to offer an advantage. Two such unconventional approaches are high frequency oscillatory ventilation (HFOV) and airway pressure release ventilation (APRV). These modes use a higher mean airway pressure (mP_{aw}) to recruit alveoli, minimize atelectrauma, and improve oxygenation. Conceptually, they appear to be ideal lung protective modes and of value in "rescue" situations, when conventional approaches fail. In this article, the authors review the principles, physiology, and the data for clinical use of HFOV and APRV in adult patients with ALI and ARDS.

High frequency oscillatory ventilation: overview and physiologic effects

The majority of clinical trials on HFOV have been performed in the neonatal population [18]. Over the past few years, coupled with better understanding of the injurious effects of mechanical ventilation, there have been renewed interest and advances in the application of HFOV in adult patients with ALI and ARDS.

HFOV is characterized by rapid oscillations of a diaphragm (in adults at frequencies of 3 Hz–10 Hz, or 180–600 breaths per minute) driven by a piston pump (Fig. 1). The forward and backward excursions of the diaphragm result in active inspiration and expiration, respectively. The pressure swings become significantly diminished as they move to the distal airways and alveoli, resulting in small V_Ts. An inspiratory bias flow (30 L–60 L per minute) and a resistance valve determine the mP_{aw} in the circuit. Unique to HFOV is the ability to decouple oxygenation and ventilation. Oxygenation is dependent on the mP_{aw} and the fraction of inspired oxygen (FiO_2). Ventilation is inversely related to the frequency and is directly related to the excursion of the diaphragm of the oscillator (pressure amplitude, ΔP). As exhalation is an active process, the risk of airtrapping or dynamic hyperinflation, at least when compared with other forms of high frequency ventilation, is reduced [19].

Gas transport is believed to occur via various mechanisms. Direct bulk flow delivers air into the alveoli situated near the proximal tracheobronchial tree. Cardiogenic oscillation and molecular diffusion aid in gas mixing. Taylor dispersion, Pendeluft effect, and asymmetric velocity profiles are the other mechanisms postulated to be involved. Detailed description of these mechanisms can be found elsewhere [19,20].

In animal studies, HFOV has been shown to be able to achieve many goals of lung protective strategy. A constant, higher mP_{aw} aids lung recruitment, maintains an open lung [21], and prevents atelectrauma. A higher mP_{aw} will also improve oxygenation and reduce the risk of oxygen toxicity. As the V_Ts delivered by HFOV are significantly lower than that of conventional ventilation, alveolar overdistension is probably mitigated. These serve to attenuate VILI, reducing the amount of histologic damage and lung inflammation [22–24].

High frequency oscillatory ventilation: clinical studies in ALI and ARDS

Current published clinical studies on the application of HFOV in adults have mainly been case series in "rescue" situations, where conventional ventilation has arguably failed. There have only been two published randomized, controlled trials where HFOV has been compared with conventional mechanical ventilation in adult ALI and ARDS. Table 1 summarizes the clinical trials on HFOV in adult ALI and ARDS subjects.

Derdak and colleagues [28] set out to compare equivalency between HFOV and conventional

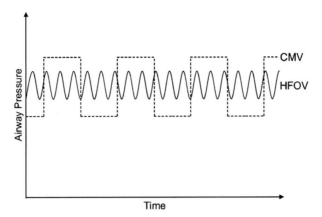

Fig. 1. Pressure-time tracing for HFOV. Pressure-time tracing for high frequency oscillatory ventilation (*solid line*) as compared with conventional mechanical ventilation (CMV) (*dashed line*). Note that frequency is not to scale. (*From* Fan E, Stewart TE. New modalities of mechanical ventilation: high frequency oscillatory ventilation and airway pressure release ventilation. Clin Chest Med 2006;27:615–25; with permission.)

ventilation (CV). In 148 subjects, key adverse events, such as oxygenation or ventilatory failure, new air leaks, intractable hypotension, and mucus plugging requiring endotracheal tube exchange were not significantly different. Interestingly, although inadequately powered, there was a nonsignificant trend toward improved 30-day mortality in those who received HFOV as compared with CV (37% versus 52%, $P = .102$). Of note, however, was that subjects in the control arm were ventilated to a V_T of up to 10 mLs/kg, the study being designed before the publication of the ARDSNet trial using smaller target V_Ts.

In the second randomized, controlled trial, involving 61 subjects [35], no significant difference was demonstrated in survival without ventilatory support or supplemental oxygen at 30 days between HFOV and CV. Methodologic problems included a need to stop the trial early because of difficulties encountered in patient recruitment, significant baseline differences in the two arms, and unequal randomization (37 subjects in the HFOV group versus 24 in the CV group). In addition, 11% of the subjects had incomplete follow-up for the primary endpoint, and 18% crossed over treatment arms during the study. The interpretation and comparison of the study results are further complicated by a lack of an explicit control arm protocol. Despite its limitations, a post hoc analysis revealed that a subgroup of subjects with the most severe hypoxemia (high oxygenation indices) tended to benefit from HFOV as compared with CV.

In a case series of 156 adult subjects with ARDS ventilated on HFOV, Mehta and colleagues [32] performed a retrospective chart review detailing the subjects'; characteristics, HFOV strategies, predictors of mortality, and outcomes. These subjects had a mean age of 48 plus or minus 18 years, mean APACHE II score of 23 plus or minus 7.5, and severe ARDS (mean PaO_2/FiO_2, 91 mm Hg plus or minus 48 mm Hg, OI 31 plus or minus 14). Significant improvement in oxygenation (PaO_2/FiO_2 and OI) was observed and sustained for a 72-hour period after the application of HFOV, although the mortality rate (61.7 %) was arguably high. Using multivariate analysis, older age, higher APACHE II score, lower pH at initiation of HFOV, and greater duration of CV before HFOV were all independent predictors of mortality. Other studies [25,27] have also illustrated that a greater number of pretreatment CV days correlated directly with mortality. This finding, however, was not confirmed in a systematic review [38].

It should be noted that the improvement in patients'; oxygenation on HFOV can be slow, in part because of small V_Ts and little tidal recruitment. The role of adjunctive therapies has been explored in several studies, with the hypothesis of additive or synergistic effects when used in combination with HFOV. The safety and efficacy of repeated RMs were demonstrated by Ferguson and colleagues [33]. Prone positioning [34] and inhaled nitric oxide [30] have also been shown to improve gas exchange in ARDS patients with sustained hypoxemia on HFOV.

Table 1
Clinical studies evaluating HFOV in adult subjects who have ALI and ARDS

Study	Study design	n	Patient population	Mortality	Comments
Fort et al [25]	Prospective observational	17	Age 38 yr PaO_2/FiO_2 69 OI 49 APACHE II 23	30-day: 53%	A greater number of pretreatment days on CMV and an OI >47 are associated with mortality. No significant compromise on cardiac output, but three subjects withdrawn from HFOV because of hypotension
Claridge et al [26]	Prospective observational	5	Trauma patients Age 37 yr PaO_2/FiO_2 52 APACHE II 29	In-hospital: 20%	HFOV used as rescue therapy for refractory hypoxemia with improvement in PaO_2/FiO_2 ratios
Mehta et al [27]	Prospective observational	24	Age 49 yr PaO_2/FiO_2 99 OI 33 APACHE II 22	30-day: 66%	No significant change in systemic BP although increases in PAOP and CVP with decrease in cardiac output noted. Pneumothoraces reported in two subjects
Derdak et al [28]	RCT	148	Age 50 yr PaO_2/FiO_2 113 OI 25 APACHE II 22	30-day HFOV: 37% CMV: 52% ($P = .102$)	No differences in hemodynamic variables, oxygenation, or ventilation failures between treatment groups. Both groups had similar complication rates
Andersen et al [29]	Retrospective	16	Age 38 yr PaO_2/FiO_2 92 OI 28 SAPS II 40	90-day: 31%	One subject had pneumothorax
Mehta et al [30]	Prospective	23	Age 45 yr PaO_2/FiO_2 75 APACHE II 29	ICU: 61%	Inhaled nitric oxide was used successfully as a viable rescue therapy in ARDS subjects on HFOV with high oxygen requirements

Study	Design	No.	Demographics	Mortality	Findings
David et al [31]	Prospective observational	42	(Median) Age 49 yr PaO_2/FiO_2 94 OI 23 APACHE II 28	30-day: 43%	Subset analysis showed subjects without oxygenation improvement after 24 hrs of HFOV had higher 30-day mortality. One subject had pneumothorax
Mehta et al [32]	Retrospective	156	(Median) Age 48 yr PaO_2/FiO_2 91 OI 31 APACHE II 24	30-day: 62%	34 subjects had a pneumothorax
Ferguson et al [33]	Prospective observational	25	(Median) Age 50 yr PaO_2/FiO_2 96 OI 23 APACHE II 24	ICU: 44%	This study demonstrated the safety and efficacy of combining lung RMs with HFOV
Papazian et al [34]	RCT	39	Age 52 yr PaO_2/FiO_2 103 SOFA 10	ICU: supine HFOV 38% prone CV 31% prone HFOV 23%	The study compared prone positioning, HFOV or their combination in ARDS subjects. Gas exchange did not improve in subjects in the supine-HFOV group. Prone position appeared superior to HFOV for oxygenation
Bollen et al [35]	RCT	61	Age 81 yr PaO_2/FiO_2 109 OI 22 APACHE II 21	30-day HFOV 43% CMV 33% ($P = .59$)	Post hoc analysis showed that a subgroup of subjects with most severe hypoxemia tended to benefit from HFOV
Pachl et al [36]	Prospective observational	30	Age 55 yr PaO_2/FiO_2 121 SOFA 10	46%	The study suggested that HFOV may benefit patients with extrapulmonary ARDS more than those with pulmonary ARDS

(continued on next page)

Table 1 (*continued*)

Study	Study design	n	Patient population	Mortality	Comments
Finkielman et al [37]	Retrospective	14	Age 56 yr PaO_2/FiO_2 73 APACHE II 35 SOFA 15	ICU: 57%	Although no change in mean arterial pressure or vasopressor requirements, one subject had HFOV withdrawn for refractory hypotension

All results reported are mean unless otherwise specified.
Abbreviations: APACHE, acute physiology and chronic health evaluation; BP, blood pressure; CMV, conventional mechanical ventilation; ICU, intensive care unit; OI, oxygenation index; PAOP, pulmonary artery occlusion pressure; RCT, randomized controlled trial; SAPS, simplified acute physiology score; SOFA, sequential organ failure assessment.

High frequency oscillatory ventilation: potential limitations and pitfalls

The higher applied $mP_{aw}s$ have invariably led to concerns of barotrauma and hemodynamic compromise. Mehta and colleagues [32] reported the incidence of pneumothorax to be 21.8%. Of 156 subjects, 26% needed to have HFOV discontinued because of problems with oxygenation and ventilation or hemodynamics. In contrast, the incidences of pneumothorax and hemodynamic instability were found to be similar in the two trials [28,35], which compared HFOV to CV. Furthermore, in 25 subjects on HFOV with an aggressive lung recruitment strategy [33], only 8% (2 subjects) required a chest tube insertion for barotrauma, and 3.3% (8 out of 244) RMs had to be aborted because of hypotension.

Recent work by Hager and colleagues [39] suggests that the V_Ts delivered by HFOV may be higher than previously thought. Data collected from seven ARDS subjects showed that V_Ts were in the range of 44 mL to 210 mL. Of particular interest, the V_Ts delivered can approach values similar to those delivered by a CV. This is especially so when HFOV is set at low frequency with a high ΔP, both of which are not uncommonly used in adult patients. By delivering V_Ts that are larger than expected, barotrauma is understandably a potential concern. Further studies are necessary to verify this finding and what impact this has on the overall goal of lung protection. At present, it may be prudent, where possible, to avoid low frequencies and high ΔP settings for adult patients on HFOV. In addition, the extent to which the higher $mP_{aw}s$ become damaging needs to be determined.

Another concern is the heavy sedation and frequent paralysis, which patients may require during HFOV. These agents can prolong duration of mechanical ventilation, lengthen ICU and hospital length of stay, and lead to complications, such as critical illness polyneuropathy [40,41].

Airway pressure release ventilation: overview and physiologic effects

APRV is a mode of ventilation designed to allow patients to breathe spontaneously while receiving high continuous positive airway pressure with an intermittent pressure release phase.

First described in 1987 [42], a continuous airway pressure (P_{high}) maintains adequate lung volumes and recruits alveoli. This, together with

FiO_2, achieves the oxygenation targets. The timing and duration of the pressure release (P_{low}) would, correspondingly, affect ventilation. The delivered V_T is, therefore, dependent on lung compliance, airway resistance, and the duration and timing of the pressure release maneuver.

The ventilator cycle essentially comprises of the inspiratory phase (during P_{high}) and the expiratory phase (during P_{low}). The patients breathe spontaneously using an active exhalation valve. These breaths can be integrated into and are independent of the ventilatory cycle (Fig. 2) [43].

In CV, V_Ts are generated by raising airway pressures above a set PEEP, potentially causing alveoli overdistension. In contrast, APRV generates V_Ts by pressure release, from P_{high} to P_{low}. As ventilation results from the decrease of pressure and lung volumes, the risk of overdistension is arguably minimized (assuming the total lung distension—caused by P_{high} plus spontaneous breaths—is in a "safe" range).

While conventional mechanically delivered breaths preferentially shift ventilation to the nondependent regions of the lungs [44], spontaneous breaths during APRV result in diaphragmatic contractions, increasing the recruitment of atelectatic alveoli in the dependent, juxtadiaphragmatic regions, improving ventilation-perfusion matching [45] and decreasing intrapulmonary shunt. Given that this is frequently a slow process, the overall improvement in oxygenation may continue over 24 hours after the start of this mode [46].

APRV may have additional physiologic benefits extending beyond ventilation and oxygenation.

The decrease in intrathoracic pressures during spontaneous breathing promotes venous return and biventricular filling, resulting in improved cardiac output and oxygen delivery [45,47]. This may result in augmented regional organ perfusion [48,49]. Given that the ability to breathe spontaneously is preserved, a unique feature of APRV is that it allows for a prolonged inspiratory phase without the need for heavy sedation and paralysis [47,50]. Intuitively, this would mean shorter ventilator days and ICU or hospital length of stay, although this finding [50] needs confirmation.

Airway pressure release ventilation: clinical studies in ALI and ARDS

There are few large clinical studies on the use of APRV in adult ALI and ARDS patients. Table 2 presents the summary of APRV trials on subjects with ALI and ARDS.

In a single center observational study on the trends in ICU mortality [56], the use of APRV was associated with a reduction in the incidence of multiorgan failure and mortality in trauma subjects with ARDS over a 2-year period, as compared with historical controls (21.4% versus 29.3%, $P<0–05$). Other modifications in therapy, such as renal replacement and vasoactive drug therapy, may also have contributed to this improvement.

In a multicenter, nonrandomized, crossover trial [51], 50 subjects with mild to moderate ALI had APRV and CMV applied sequentially for 30 minutes. Similar oxygenation and

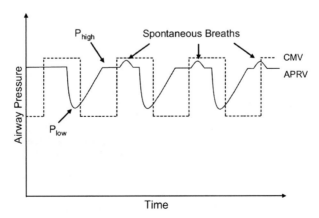

Fig. 2. Pressure-time tracing for APRV. Pressure-time tracing for airway pressure release ventilation (*solid line*) as compared with conventional mechanical ventilation (*dashed line*). (*From* Fan E, Stewart TE. New modalities of mechanical ventilation: high frequency oscillatory ventilation and airway pressure release ventilation. Clin Chest Med 2006;27: 615–25; with permission.)

Table 2
Clinical studies evaluating APRV in adult subjects who have ALI and ARDS

Study	Study design	N	Patient population	Mortality	Comments
Rasanen et al [51]	Prospective crossover trial	50	Age 47 yr Medical patients, acute respiratory failure	In-hospital: 30%	Subjects on APRV had significant reduction in peak airway pressures
Davis et al [52]	Prospective crossover trial	15	Trauma patients with ARDS	Not reported	Lower PIP and PEEP. There was no difference in gas exchange and hemodynamic variables
Sydow et al [46]	RCT	18	Age 53 yr PaO_2/FiO_2 140 LIS 2.3	In-hospital: 22%	Lower PIP with better oxygenation and improved venous admixture
Putensen et al [50]	RCT	30	Trauma patients Age 41 yr PaO_2/FiO_2 245 SAPS 18	In-hospital APRV 20% CMV 26%	Ventilator and ICU days shorter with APRV. Better gas exchange and better hemodynamics. Less need for sedation and vasopressors
Varpula et al [54]	RCT	45	(Median) Age 48 yr PaO_2/FiO_2 130 APACHE II 14	28-day APRV 8% CMV 14%	Prone position shown to be feasible in APRV with improvement in PaO_2/FiO_2 ratio after 24 hours
Varpula et al [53]	RCT	58	(Median) Age 47 yr PaO_2/FiO_2 157 APACHE II 15	28-day APRV 17% CMV 18%	No difference in ventilator-free days at day 28
Dart et al [55]	Retrospective	46	Trauma patients PaO_2/FiO_2 243	Not reported	APRV is a safe alternative. Improved PaO_2/FiO_2 ratio with decreased peak airway pressures at 72 hours

All results reported are mean unless otherwise specified.
Abbreviations: LIS, lung injury score; PIP, peak inspiratory pressure.

hemodynamic goals were achieved. Although the mP_{aw} during either of the ventilatory modes were comparable, there was a significant decrease in the peak airway pressures (55 plus or minus 17%, $P < .0001$) while the subjects were on APRV as compared with CV. The study, however, lacked a rigorous study design and without an explicit lung protective strategy protocol (during CV), the extrapolation of these results into clinical practice is difficult.

Putensen and colleagues [50] assessed the cardiorespiratory function in 30 trauma subjects who had or were at risk of ALI. The subjects were randomized to APRV or pressure controlled ventilation (PCV). Improved cardiac index with significantly lower systemic and pulmonary vascular resistance were found in the APRV group. Despite similar hemodynamic targets, the amount of vasopressors or inotropic support was lower in patients with APRV. There were also encouraging

secondary outcomes from this study. The durations of ventilatory support (15 versus 21 days, $P = .032$), intubation (18 versus 25 days, $P = .011$), and length of ICU stay (23 versus 30 days, $P = .032$) were shorter in the APRV group as compared with CV. However, the significance of these findings is debatable, as patients randomized to the PCV group were, initially, paralyzed for 72 hours.

In the largest published randomized, controlled trial, Varpula and colleagues [53] compared APRV to synchronized intermittent ventilation with pressure control or pressure support (SIMV-PC/PS) in a single center. The study was terminated early for futility after recruiting 58 (out of a target of 80) subjects. There were no significant baseline characteristic differences between the two groups of subjects. The majority had primary ALI (77%) and the median duration of mechanical ventilation before randomization was 39.1 plus or minus 2.3 hours. Although inspiratory pressures were lower (25.9 cm H_2O plus or minus 0.6 cm H_2O versus 28.6 cm H_2O plus or minus 0.7 cm H_2O , $P = .007$) in the APRV group during the first week, other physiologic parameters (PaO_2/FiO_2, pH, $PaCO_2$, minute ventilation, mean arterial pressure, cardiac output) were comparable between the two arms. At 28 days, there were no statistical differences in the number of ventilator-free days after randomization between APRV and SIMV-PC/PS (13.4 plus or minus 1.7 days versus 12.2 plus or minus 1.5 days, $P = .83$). Mortality at 28 days (17% versus 18%, respectively, $P = .91$) and at 1 year (17% versus 25%, $P = .43$) were similar as well. As the trial was designed before the publication of ARDSNet [16], both the intervention and control arms had the driving pressure titrated to achieve 8 mL/kg–10 mL/kg V_T. What impact this has on the overall outcomes remains unclear.

Airway pressure release ventilation: potential limitations and pitfalls

There are theoretic risks of VILI during APRV. It is important to note that the set P_{high} is not necessarily the maximal stretching pressure to which the lungs are subjected. Spontaneous breathing during P_{high} generates negative pleural pressures that add to the stretch. This has to be considered when evaluating the maximal stretch to which the lungs are exposed. Neumann and colleagues [43] demonstrated aggregate tidal volumes approaching 1 L in airway pressure, flow, and volume tracings. In addition, shearing and atelectrauma need to be considered when the ventilator cycling between P_{high} to P_{low} occurs.

Despite these potential limitations—which is not unique to APRV—a reduced need for sedation and analgesia would make APRV an attractive ventilatory mode. This theoretic benefit, although encouraging, has not been proven conclusively, as clinical trials to date have shown conflicting results [47,50,54].

Discussion

HFOV and APRV are unique "open lung" ventilatory strategies which may offer improved gas exchange and lung protection. Their favorable physiologic effects, however, have not been translated into demonstrable survival benefits in clinical trials. It is important to note that improved physiology (for instance improved oxygenation) does not necessarily translate into improved outcome. For example, patients ventilated in the small tidal volume arm of the ARDSNet [16] protocol had an early worsening of oxygenation, but had significant reduction in mortality. Consistent with this idea, it is important to note that patients with ALI and ARDS who do not survive, infrequently die as a result of hypoxemia, compared with multisystem organ failure. At present, widespread adoption of HFOV and APRV is difficult to recommend in the absence of data showing these modes to be superior to the optimal lung-protective conventional ventilation. For now, their utility appears to be in situations where patients have failed conventional mechanical ventilation.

Future research on HFOV and APRV should strive to identify the ideal patient population who would benefit most, the timing, as well as the best way to deliver these ventilatory modes. At this point, the authors are aware of an ongoing large international multicenter randomized, controlled trial comparing HFOV to optimal lung protective conventional ventilation (M. Meade and N. Ferguson, personal communication, 2007: Oscillate Trial) which we anticipate will help clarify the role of HFOV and provide further directions in its clinical application.

The dilemma faced by intensivists today when deciding what to do with therapies largely proven in "rescue" situations, is best highlighted by Smith and Pell [57]. To determine the effectiveness of parachutes in skydivers, Smith and his coauthor attempted, without success, a systematic review of randomized controlled trials on their use. Obviously, no one had attempted an RCT involving the use of a parachute when skydiving. The investigators had no choice but to conclude that, at times, it is appropriate to use certain rescue therapies despite the absence of a high level RCT. Such may be the case for HFOV and APRV.

References

[1] Rubenfeld GD, Caldwell E, Peabody E, et al. Incidence and outcomes of acute lung injury. N Engl J Med 2005;353:1685–93.

[2] Goss CH, Brower RG, Hudson LD, et al. Incidence of acute lung injury in the United States. Crit Care Med 2003;31:1607–11.

[3] Luhr OR, Antonsen K, Karlsson M, et al. Incidence and mortality after acute respiratory failure and acute respiratory distress syndrome in Sweden, Denmark and Iceland. The ARF study group. Am J Respir Crit Care Med 1999;159:1849–61.

[4] Rubenfeld GD, Herridge MS. Epidemiology and outcomes of acute lung injury. Chest 2007;131:554–62.

[5] Wheeler AP, Bernard GR. Acute lung injury and the acute respiratory distress syndrome: a clinical review. Lancet 2007;369:1553–65.

[6] American Thoracic Society. International consensus conferences in intensive care medicine: ventilator associated lung injury in ARDS. Am J Respir Crit Care Med 1999;160(18):2118–24.

[7] Plotz FB, Slutsky AS, van Vught AJ, et al. Ventilator induced lung injury and multiple system organ failure: a critical review of facts and hypotheses. Intensive Care Med 2004;30:1865–72.

[8] Ranieri VM, Suter PM, Tortorella C, et al. Effect of mechanical ventilation on inflammatory mediators in patients with acute respiratory distress syndrome. A randomized controlled trial. JAMA 1999;282: 54–61.

[9] Slutsky AS, Tremblay LN. Multiple system organ failure. Is mechanical ventilation a contributing factor? Am J Respir Crit Care Med 1998;157:1721–5.

[10] Carmichael LC, Dorinskey PM, Higgins SB, et al. Diagnosis and therapy of cute respiratory syndrome in adults: an international survey. J Crit Care 1996; 11:9–18.

[11] Chonghaile MN, Higgins B, Laffey JG. Permissive hypercapnia: role in protective lung ventilation strategies. Curr Opin Crit Care 2005;11:56–62.

[12] Amato MBP, Barbas CSV, Medeiros DM, et al. Effect of a protective-ventilation strategy on mortality in the acute respiratory distress syndrome. N Engl J Med 1998;338:347–54.

[13] Villar J, Kacmarek RM, Perez-Mendez L, et al. A high positive end-expiratory pressure, low tidal volume ventilatory strategy improves outcome in persistent acute respiratory distress syndrome: a randomized, controlled trial. Crit Care Med 2006;34(5): 1311–8.

[14] Meade MO, Cook DJ, Guyatt GH, et al. Ventilatory strategy using low tidal volumes, recruitment maneuvres and high positive end expiratory pressure for acute lung injury and acute respiratory distress syndrome. A randomized controlled trial. JAMA 2008;299(6):637–45.

[15] Mercat A, Richard JC, Vielle B, et al. Positive end expiratory pressure setting in adults with acute lung injury and acute respiratory distress syndrome. A randomized controlled trial. JAMA 2008;299(6): 646–55.

[16] The Acute Respiratory Distress Syndrome Network. Ventilation with lower tidal volumes as compared with traditional tidal volumes for acute lung injury and the acute respiratory distress syndrome. N Engl J Med 2000;342:1301–8.

[17] Terragni PP, Rosboch G, Tealdi A, et al. Tidal hyperinflation during low tidal volume ventilation in acute respiratory distress syndrome. Am J Respir Crit Care Med 2007;175:160–6.

[18] Froese AB, Kineslla JP. High frequency oscillatory ventilation: lessons from the neonatal/pediatric experience. Crit Care Med 2005;33:S115–21.

[19] Krishnan JA, Brower RC. High-frquency ventilation for acute lung injury and ARDS. Chest 2000; 118:795–807.

[20] Slutsky AS, Drazen JM. Ventilation with small tidal volumes. N Engl J Med 2002;347:630–1.

[21] Hamilton PP, Onayemi A, Smyth JA, et al. Comparison of conventional and high frequency ventilation: oxygenation and lung pathology. J Appl Physiol 1983;55:131–8.

[22] Imai Y, Nakagawa S, Ito Y, et al. Comparison of lung protection strategies using conventional and high frequency oscillatory ventilation. J Appl Physiol 2001;91:1836–44.

[23] Rotta AT, Gunnarsson B, Fuhrman BP, et al. Comparison of lung protective ventilation strategies in a rabbit model of acute lung injury. Crit Care Med 2001;29:2176–84.

[24] Muellenbach RM, Kredel M, Said HM, et al. High frequency ventilation reduces lung inflammation: a large-animal 24-h model of respiratory distress. Intensive Care Med 2007;33:1423–33.

[25] Fort P, Farmer C, Westerman J, et al. High-frequency oscillatory ventilation for adult respiratory distress syndrome: a pilot study. Crit Care Med 1997;25:937–47.

[26] Claridge JA, Hostetter RG, Lowson SM, et al. High-frequency oscillatory ventilation can be effective as rescue therapy for refractory acute lung dysfunction. Am Surg 1999;65:1092–6.

[27] Mehta S, Lapinsky SE, Hallet DC, et al. Prospective trial of high-frequency oscillation in adults with acute respiratory distress syndrome. Crit Care Med 2001;29:1360–9.

[28] Derdak S, Mehta S, Stewart TE, et al. High-frequency oscillatory ventilation for acute respiratory distress syndrome in adults: a randomized, controlled trial. Am J Respir Crit Care Med 2002; 166:801–8.

[29] Andersen FA, Guttormsen AB, Flaaten HK. High-frequency oscillatory ventilation in adult patients with acute respiratory distress syndrome: a retrospective study. Acta Anaesthesiol Scand 2002;46: 1082–8.

[30] Mehta S, Macdonald R, Hallet DC, et al. Acute oxygenation response to inhaled nitric oxide when combined with high-frequency oscillatory ventilation in adults with acute respiratory distress syndrome. Crit Care Med 2003;31:383–9.

[31] David M, Weiler N, Heinrichs W, et al. High-frequency oscillatory ventilation in adult acute respiratory distress syndrome. Intensive Care Med 2003;29:1656–65.

[32] Mehta S, Granton J, MacDonald RJ, et al. High-frequency oscillatory ventilation in adults: the Toronto experience. Chest 2004;126:518–27.

[33] Ferguson ND, Chiche JD, Kacmarek RM, et al. Combining high-frequency oscillatory ventilation and recruitment maneuvers in adults with early acute respiratory distress syndrome: the treatment with oscillation and an open lung strategy (TOOLS) trial pilot study. Crit Care Med 2005; 33:479–86.

[34] Papazian L, Gainnier M, Martin V, et al. Comaprison of prone positioning and high-frequency oscillatory ventilation in patients with acute respiratory distress syndrome. Crit Care Med 2005;33: 2162–71.

[35] Bollen CW, van Well GT, Sherry T, et al. High-frequency oscillatory ventilation compared with conventional mechanical ventilation in adult respiratory distress syndrome: a randomized controlled trial. Crit Care 2005;9:430–9.

[36] Pachl J, Roubik K, Waldauf P, et al. Normocapnic high-frequency oscillatory ventilation affects differently extrapulmonary and pulmonary forms of acute respiratory distress syndrome in adults. Physiol Res 2006;55:15–24.

[37] Finkielman JD, Gajic O, Farmer JC, et al. The initial mayo clinic experience using high-frequency oscillatory ventilation for adult patients: a retrospective study. BMC Emerg Med 2006;6:2.

[38] Bollen CW, Uiterwaal CS, van Vught AJ. Systematic review of determinants of mortality in high frequency oscillatory ventilation in acute respiratory distress syndrome. Crit Care 2006;10:R34.

[39] Hager DN, Fessler HE, Kaczka DW, et al. Tidal volume delivery during high-frequency oscillatory ventilation in adults with acute respiratory distress syndrome. Crit Care Med 2007;35:1522–9.

[40] Kress JP, Pohlman AS, O'Connor MF, et al. Daily interruption of sedative infusion in critically ill patients undergoing mechanical ventilation. N Engl J Med 2000;342:1471–7.

[41] Latronico N, Peli E, Botteri M. Critical illness myopathy and neuropathy. Curr Opin Crit Care 2005;11:126–32.

[42] Stock MC, Downs JB, Frolicher DA. Airway pressure release ventilation. Crit Care Med 1987; 15:462–6.

[43] Neumann P, Golisch W, Stromeyer A, et al. Influence of different release times on spontaneous breathing during airway pressure release ventilation. Intensive Care Med 2002;28:1742–9.

[44] Reber A, Nylund U, Hedenstierna G. Position and shape of the diaphragm: implications for atelectasis formation. Anaesthesia 1998;53:1054–61.

[45] Putensen C, Mutz NJ, Putensen-Himmer G, et al. Spontaneous breathing during ventilatory support improves ventilation-prefusion distributions in patients with acute respiratory distress syndrome. Am J Respir Crit Care Med 1999;159:1241–8.

[46] Sydow M, Burchardi H, Ephraim E, et al. Long-term effects of two different ventilatory modes on oxygenation in acute lung injury: comparison of airway pressure release ventilation and volume-controlled inverse ratio ventilation. Am J Respir Crit Care Med 1994;149:1550–6.

[47] Kaplan LJ, Bailey H, Formosa V. Airway pressure release ventilation increases cardiac performance in patients with acute lung injury/adult respiratory distress syndrome. Crit Care 2001;5:221–6.

[48] Hering R, Peters D, Zinserling J, et al. Effects of spontaneous breathing during airway pressure release ventilation on renal perfusion and function in patients with acute lung injury. Intensive Care Med 2002;28:1426–33.

[49] Hering R, Viehofer A, Zinserling J, et al. Effects of spontaneous breathing during airway pressure release ventilation on intestinal blood flow in experimental lung injury. Anesthesiology 2003;99:1137–44.

[50] Putensen C, Zech S, Wriggle H, et al. Long term effects of spontaneous breathing during ventilatory support in patients with acute lung injury. Am J Respir Crit Care Med 2001;164:43–9.

[51] Rasanen J, Cane RD, Downs JB, et al. Airway pressure release ventilation during acute lung injury: a prospective multicenter trial. Crit Care Med 1991; 19:1234–41.

[52] Davis K, Johnson DJ, Branson RD, et al. Airway pressure release ventilation. Arch Surg 1993;128: 1348–52.

[53] Varpula T, Valta P, Niemi R, et al. Airway pressure release ventilation as a primary ventilatory mode in acute respiratory distress syndrome. Acta Anaesthesiol Scand 2004;48:722–31.

[54] Varpula T, Jousela I, Niemi R, et al. Combined effects of prone positioning and airway pressure release ventilation on gas exchange in patients with acute lung injury. Acta Anaesthesiol Scand 2003; 47:516–24.

[55] Dart BW, Maxwell RA, Richart CM, et al. Preliminary experience with airway pressure release ventilation in a trauma/surgical intensive care unit. J Trauma 2005;59:71–6.

[56] Navarrete-Navarra P, Rodriguez A, Reynolds H, et al. Acute respiratory distress syndrome among trauma patients: trends in ICU mortality, risk factors, complications and resource utilization. Intensive Care Med 2001;27:1133–40.

[57] Smith GCS, Pell JP. Parachute use to prevent death and major trauma related to gravitational challenge: systematic review of randomized controlled trials. BMJ 2003;327:1459–61.

ELSEVIER
SAUNDERS

Clin Chest Med 29 (2008) 277–296

CLINICS
IN CHEST
MEDICINE

How Best to Deliver Aerosol Medications to Mechanically Ventilated Patients

Rajiv Dhand, MD[a,b,c,*], Vamsi P. Guntur, MD[a,c]

[a]Division of Pulmonary, Critical Care, and Environmental Medicine, University of Missouri,
MA-421 Health Sciences Center, 1 Hospital Drive, Columbia, MO 65212, USA
[b]Harry S. Truman Veterans' Affairs Hospital, 800 Hospital Drive, Columbia, MO 65201, USA
[c]University of Missouri Hospitals and Clinics, 1 Hospital Drive, Columbia, MO 65212, USA

In intubated and mechanically ventilated patients, the presence of an artificial airway significantly reduces the efficiency of aerosolized therapy: that is, the proportion of the nominal dose that is delivered to the lung. MacIntyre and colleagues [1] published a landmark study showing that pulmonary deposition of a radio-labeled aerosol in mechanically ventilated patients was much lower than that previously noted in ambulatory patients. Likewise, Fuller and colleagues [2] performed a comparison study in mechanically ventilated patients and found that the efficiency of drug delivery with both pressurized metered-dose inhalers (pMDIs) and nebulizers was lower than that achieved in ambulatory patients. In 1991, a consensus statement by experts convened by the American Association of Respiratory Care pointed out the lack of information about the best techniques for delivering aerosols in ventilator-supported patients [3]. Over the following 25 years, knowledge about aerosol delivery in patients receiving mechanical ventilation has evolved rapidly, and there is now a much greater understanding of the scientific basis for aerosol therapy in this patient population [4–6]. In fact, with improvement in techniques for aerosol delivery and with development of newer aerosol generators, the efficiency of aerosol delivery in patients receiving mechanical ventilation has improved to a level that matches and may even surpass that reported in spontaneously breathing patients [7].

How should aerosols be administered to mechanically ventilated patients? This is an important question because aerosol administration to mechanically ventilated patients differs in important respects from the techniques employed in ambulatory patients (Table 1). Moreover, variations in the technique of administration lead to marked differences in the amount of drug delivered to the lower respiratory tract [4,5]. For example, Manthous and colleagues [8] found no response in up to 100 puffs of albuterol (10 mg) with a pMDI, whereas there was a significant reduction in airway resistance with 2.5 mg of albuterol administered with a jet nebulizer. This lack of effect with pMDIs was attributed to the poor efficiency of the elbow adapter employed in this study [9], such that most of the drug from the pMDI was probably deposited in the actuator or endotracheal tube and negligible amounts were delivered to the patients' airways. Subsequently, several investigators found significant bronchodilator responses with administration of albuterol by a pMDI and chamber spacer [10–19]. Thus, optimal aerosol delivery requires careful consideration of several factors that influence aerosol delivery to the lungs of patients receiving mechanical ventilation.

A host of factors influence the efficiency of drug delivery during mechanical ventilation (Fig. 1). The major factors that need to be

This work was supported by the Veterans' Affairs Research Service.

* Corresponding author. Division of Pulmonary, Critical Care, Environmental Medicine, University of Missouri, MA-421 Health Sciences Center, 1 Hospital Drive, Columbia, MO 65212.

E-mail address: dhandr@health.missouri.edu (R. Dhand).

0272-5231/08/$ - see front matter. Published by Elsevier Inc.
doi:10.1016/j.ccm.2008.02.003

Table 1
Differences in aerosol delivery in spontaneously breathing versus mechanically ventilated patients

	Spontaneously breathing patient	Mechanically ventilated patient
Position of the patient	Sitting or standing	Laying supine or semi-recumbent
Aerosol-generator	pMDI/pMDI and spacer/dry powder inhaler/nebulizer	pMDI and spacer/nebulizer
Method of delivery	By mouthpiece or facemask	Connected to endotracheal tube or inspiratory limb of ventilator circuit
Humidity	Ambient humidity	Humidifed (approximately 97% relative humidity)
Temperature	Room or ambient	Warmed to approximately 35°C
Inspiratory airflow	Sinusoidal	Constant or ramp flow
Breath configuration	Controlled by patient	Controlled by ventilator[a]
Aerosol administration	Self-administered	Administered by nurse or therapist
Airway	Oral or nasal cavity and upper airway	Artificial airway

[a] In controlled modes of mechanical ventilation, the ventilator controls the breath configuration. In assisted modes of ventilation, the breath configuration is influenced by the patient's effort.

considered include: (1) the position of the patient; (2) the aerosol generator and its configuration in the ventilator circuit; (3) aerosol particle size; (4) synchronization of aerosol generation with inspiratory airflow from the ventilator; (5) conditions in the ventilator circuit; and (6) ventilatory parameters [5,6,20]. Other factors that influence the response to aerosolized therapy are the dose of the drug, the duration of action, and certain patient characteristics, such as the presence of airflow obstruction or dynamic hyperinflation (see Fig. 1) [11,12,19]. Monitoring the response

Ventilator-related
• Ventilation mode
• Tidal volume
• Respiratory rate
• Duty cycle
• Inspiratory waveform
• Breath-triggering mechanism

Device-related - MDI
• Type of spacer or adapter
• Position of spacer in circuit
• Timing of MDI actuation
• Type of MDI

Drug-related
• Dose
• Formulation
• Aerosol particle size
• Targeted site for delivery
• Duration of action

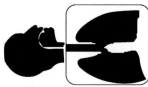

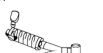

Device-related - nebulizer
• Type of nebulizer
• Fill volume
• Gas flow
• Cycling: inspiration vs continuous
• Duration of nebulization
• Position in the circuit

Patient-related
• Severity of airway obstruction
• Mechanism of airway obstruction
• Presence of dynamic hyperinflation
• Patient-ventilator synchrony

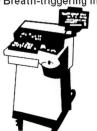

Circuit-related
• Endotracheal tube size
• Humidity of inhaled gas
• Density of inhaled gas

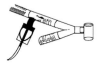

Fig. 1. Aerosol delivery in mechanically ventilated patients is complex. Careful attention to a host of factors, including the position of the patient, the type of aerosol generator and its configuration in the ventilator circuit, aerosol particle size, the type and size of the artificial airway, conditions in the ventilator circuit (such as humidity and density of the carrier gas), and ventilatory parameters, is needed to optimize aerosol delivery during mechanical ventilation. MDI, metered-dose inhaler. (*From* Dhand R. Basic techniques for aerosol delivery during mechanical ventilation. Respir Care 2004;49:611–22; with permission.)

to treatment can also differ between intubated and nonintubated patients [11,12,19,21,22].

Position of the patient

Spontaneously breathing patients usually adopt a sitting or standing posture during aerosol inhalation. In contrast, most patients are recumbent or semi-recumbent while receiving mechanical ventilation and inhaled drug therapy. Ventilator-dependent patients should preferably sit in bed or in a chair during inhalation therapy. In patients with acute exacerbations of chronic obstructive pulmonary disease (COPD), administration of bronchodilator aerosols to semi-recumbent patients produced a significant response [11,12,14,15,17,19]. A semi-recumbent position, with the head end of the bed elevated to 20 to 30 degrees above horizontal, should suffice for ventilator-supported patients who are unable to sit erect during aerosol administration.

The aerosol generator

In ambulatory patients, pMDIs, nebulizers, and dry powder inhalers are the aerosol-generating devices of choice for inhalation therapy. Similarly to ambulatory patients, aerosol delivery during mechanical ventilation also depends to a great extent on the type of aerosol-generating device employed; however, only pMDIs and nebulizers have been adapted for clinical use during mechanical ventilation [6]. A variety of drugs or therapeutic agents could be delivered to the lung by inhalation (Box 1). The techniques for using

pMDIs differ from those employed for nebulizers and these devices are discussed separately.

pMDIs

In mechanically ventilated patients, pMDIs are chiefly used to deliver beta-adrenergic and anticholinergic bronchodilators for treatment of airway obstruction [4–6,23]. Within the past decade, pMDIs have become more popular than nebulizers for routine bronchodilator therapy in the intensive care unit (ICU).

Chlorofluorocarbon versus hydrofluoroalkane-pMDIs

Previously, most pMDIs used chlorofluorocarbon (CFC) propellants, but these are being phased out and will be largely replaced by a newer generation of pMDIs containing hydrofluoroalkane (HFA) propellants [24]. In the United States, full transition from CFC to HFA-pMDIs is scheduled for the end of 2008 [25], but will probably occur sooner for short-acting bronchodilator aerosols. Most of the CFC-pMDIs were suspensions of drug powder in surfactant [26]. Preservatives and antioxidants were added to improve the shelf-life of the inhaler. The initial albuterol sulfate HFA-pMDI (Airomir, 3M Pharmaceuticals, St Paul, Minnesota), a suspension formulation containing a low concentration of ethanol, had aerosol characteristics and clinical responses similar to those observed with the albuterol CFC-pMDI [27]. Because HFA-propellants are not compatible with surfactants [28], the newer HFA-pMDIs have been reformulated as ethanolic solutions, resulting in a finer aerosol spray [29–31]

Box 1. Inhaled medications employed in patients receiving mechanical ventilation

Bronchodilator
    Beta-agonist (albuterol, metaproteronol, fenoterol)
    Anticholinergic (ipratropium bromide)
Prostaglandin (alprostadil, prostacyclin, iloprost, treprostonil)
Mucolytics (acetylcysteine)
Proteins (Pulmozyme)
Surfactant (Exosurf)
Antibiotics
Antibacterial (aminoglycosides)
Antiviral (Ribavirin)
Antifungal (amphotericin)
Corticosteroids (beclomethasone; budesonide)
Miscellaneous

with greater peripheral lung deposition and improved efficacy when compared with the CFC-pMDIs [32,33]. In contrast to the albuterol base in most CFC-pMDIs, the newer albuterol HFA-pMDIs contain albuterol sulfate. Table 2 shows the constituents of currently available albuterol pMDIs [34,35].

Despite differences in the pMDI formulation, clinical effects of albuterol HFA-pMDIs are similar to those of albuterol CFC-pMDIs. In both adults [36] and children [37] with asthma, the bronchodilator responses to administration of albuterol HFA-pMDIs were similar to those obtained with albuterol CFC-pMDIs. Patients with asthma who were on regular treatment with albuterol CFC-pMDI could be switched to regular treatment with HFA-pMDIs without any deterioration in pulmonary function or loss of asthma control [38,39]. Likewise, the albuterol HFA-pMDI was equally effective as a CFC-pMDI in protecting against methacholine-induced bronchoconstriction [40]. Long-term postapproval studies found that asthma control in subjects randomized to receive albuterol HFA-pMDI were similar to that in those receiving albuterol CFC-pMDI [41,42]. After-marketing surveillance studies in the United Kingdom that enrolled over 17,000 subjects in an open-label study found no difference in hospital admissions or unusual adverse events between subjects receiving albuterol CFC- or HFA-pMDIs [43,44]. In normal subjects, self-administration of HFA propellant for 28 days produced lesser side effects than the use of a CFC propellant [45]. In clinical trials in children and adults, the frequency of adverse events with the use of HFA albuterol were similar to those with CFC albuterol [24]. Tremor, nervousness, headache, and tachycardia were the most frequently reported side effects, but they were each observed in less than 10% of patients using albuterol HFA-pMDIs [24].

Spacer or adapter devices

Several commercially available adapters or actuators are used to connect the pMDI canister to the ventilator circuit. The type of adapter employed could have a profound influence on the efficiency of drug delivery [4–6,9,23,46]. The types of adapters available for clinical use include elbow adapters, inline devices that may be unidirectional or bidirectional, and chamber or reservoir adapters (Fig. 2) [4–6,9,23]. A chamber spacer with a pMDI in a ventilator circuit results in four- to sixfold greater aerosol drug delivery, compared with either an elbow adapter or

Table 2
Metered-dose inhalers containing albuterol that are approved for use in the United States

Propellant	Type	Contents	μg/puff (total doses)	Contents	Remarks
CFC[a]	suspension	Albuterol base	90 (200)	Oleic acid	Prime after 4 days[g]
CFC[b]	suspension	Albuterol sulfate/ Ipratropium bromide	90 (200) 18	Soya lecithin	Prime after 24 hours[g]
HFA[c]	solution	Albuterol sulfate	90 of base (200)	Ethanol	Prime after 2 weeks[g]
HFA[d]	solution	Albuterol sulfate	90 of base (200)	Ethanol + oleic acid	Prime after 2 weeks[g]
HFA[e]	solution	Albuterol sulfate	90 of base (200)	No excipient[h]	Prime after 2 weeks[g]
HFA[f]	solution	Levalbuterol tartarate	45 of base (200)	Ethanol + oleic acid	Prime after 3 days[g]

[a] Generic albuterol, manufactured by Armstrong Pharmaceuticals, West Roxbury, Massachusetts.

[b] Combivent, manufactured by Boehringer-Ingelheim, Ridgefield, Connecticut.

[c] ProAir HFA, manufactured by IVAX Laboratories, Miami, Florida.

[d] Proventil HFA, manufactured by Schering-Plough, Kenilworth, New Jersey.

[e] Ventolin HFA, manufactured by GlaxoSmithKline, Research Triangle Park, North Carolina.

[f] Xopenex HFA, manufactured by Sepracor, Marlborough, Massachusetts.

[g] Contents may leak from the metering chamber when the inhaler has not been used for some time. This may result in delivery of an inadequate dose. Recommend to prime by actuating 4 puffs before the first use or when the inhaler has not been used for the specified period [34].

[h] HFA propellants have higher moisture affinity than CFCs [35]. Thus, water may seep around the gaskets in the metering-valve into the canister. Ventolin-HFA has a shorter shelf life and should be discarded 2 months after it is removed from the pouch.

Data from Hendeles L, Colice GL, Meyer RJ. Withdrawal of albuterol inhalers containing chlorofluorocarbon propellants. N Engl J Med 2007;356:1344–51.

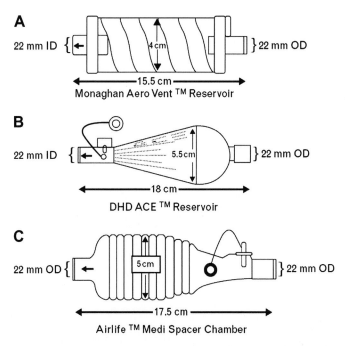

Fig. 2. A variety of chamber spacers are used to connect a metered-dose inhaler canister in the ventilator circuit. (*A*) Collapsible spacer chamber; (*B*) aerosol cloud enhancer, wherein the aerosol flume is directed away from the patient; (*C*) noncollapsible spacer chamber. (*Adapted from* Rau JL, Dunlevy CL, Hill RL. A comparison of inline MDI actuators for delivery of a beta agonist and a corticosteroid with a mechanically-ventilated lung model. Respir Care 1998;43: 705–12; with permission.)

a unidirectional inline spacer [9,47–49]. A pMDI and chamber spacer placed at a distance of approximately 15 cm from the endotracheal tube provides efficient aerosol delivery and elicits a significant bronchodilator response [11,12]. Rau and colleagues [50] found that the efficiency of a bidirectional inline spacer was higher than a unidirectional inline spacer and was comparable to that achieved with chamber spacers [50]; however, the performance of the bidirectional spacer has not been established in clinical studies.

To improve drug delivery with HFA-pMDIs in the setting of mechanical ventilation, the actuators required to connect them in ventilator circuits need to be matched to the size of the pMDI canister stem [51]. No commercially available actuator is equally efficient with all pMDIs, and HFA-pMDIs will need to be matched with suitable actuators to optimize their efficiency during mechanical ventilation. Because the plume from a HFA-pMDI is smaller and less forceful than that from a CFC-pMDI, less drug is expected to deposit on the walls of the spacer [30,52,53]. However, in bench models of mechanical ventilation, albuterol HFA-pMDIs employed with an

Aerovent spacer (Monaghan Medical, Plattsburgh, New York) provided drug delivery that was lower than that with CFC-pMDIs [51]. Contrarily, beclomethasone HFA-pMDIs employed with an Aerochamber HC MV spacer (Monaghan Medical, Plattsburgh, New York) (Fig. 3) had a higher efficiency of drug delivery than the beclomethasone CFC-pMDI [54]. The differences in the results of the studies could be explained by differences in the pMDI formulation and types of spacers employed by the two groups of investigators. The beclomethasone HFA-pMDI is formulated as a solution and produces an extra fine aerosol with mass median aerodynamic diameter (MMAD) of 1.2 μm, whereas the albuterol HFA-pMDI was a suspension with aerosol particle size comparable to that of the albuterol CFC-pMDI. Moreover, the size of the canister stem is different for each pMDI and the efficiency of drug delivery depends on how well the canister stem fits into the actuator (Table 3) [51]. Therefore, the differences in the results of the two studies could also be because of the different spacers employed by the investigators (Aerovent versus Aerochamber HC MV). In a neonatal lung model

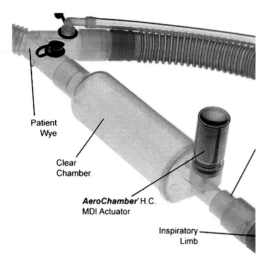

Patient
Wye

Clear
Chamber

AeroChamber H.C.
MDI Actuator

Inspiratory
Limb

Fig. 3. The Aerochamber HC MV is designed for use during mechanical ventilation. The see-through chamber allows observation of the aerosol spray. It could be employed with HFA-pMDIs. It can be placed in the inspiratory limb of the ventilator circuit (as shown) or it could be connected directly to an endotracheal or tracheostomy tube. (*Courtesy of* Trudell Medical International, London, ON; with permission.)

of mechanical ventilation, no differences in drug delivery were observed between CFC- and HFA-pMDIs with regard to drug delivery [55,56].

In summary, significant changes have been made in the formulation and characteristics of HFA- compared with CFC-pMDIs. The clinical

Table 3
Effect of actuator and nozzle size on drug output and aerosol particle size

Canister	Actuator	MMAD ± GSD	Total mass (g/m^2)
CFC	CFC	2.51 ± 2.8	3.5
CFC	HFA	1.32 ± 3.1[a]	1.7[a]
HFA	HFA	2.16 ± 2.3	4.4
HFA	CFC	4.59 ± 4.2	1.2
CFC	Adapter	2.12 ± 1.9	2.1
HFA	Adapter	3.52 ± 3.1[a]	1.1[a]

Abbreviations: Adapter, a standard adapter employed in ventilator circuits; GSD, geometric standard deviation.

[a] $P < .001$ compared with CFC pMDI and standard actuator.

Data from Fink JB, Dhand R, Grychowski J, et al. Reconciling in-vitro and in-vivo measurements of aerosol delivery from a metered-dose inhaler during mechanical ventilation, and defining efficiency enhancing factors. Am J Respir Crit Care Med 1999;159:63–8.

implications of these changes for spontaneously breathing, ambulatory patients are shown in Table 4 [29–31,34,57–65]. In ventilator-supported patients, transition to HFA-pMDIs is likely to have a major influence on drug delivery and response to treatment with pMDIs. However, to the best of the authors' knowledge, the optimal methods to administer albuterol HFA-pMDIs and the response to drug administration have not been investigated in mechanically ventilated patients.

Nebulizers

Both jet and ultrasonic nebulizers have been employed for aerosol delivery during mechanical ventilation. Nebulizers are employed to deliver a variety of agents, such as bronchodilators, prostanoids, antibiotics, surfactant, mucolytic agents, and corticosteroids to mechanically ventilated patients (see Box 1) [66–68].

Jet nebulizers

During mechanical ventilation, jet nebulizers are connected in the inspiratory limb of the ventilator circuit and may be operated continuously by pressurized gas from a wall system or gas cylinder, or intermittently by using a separate line to provide driving pressure and gas flow from the ventilator. During intermittent operation, the nebulizer generates aerosol only during the inspiratory phase, and the ventilator compensates for the flow to the nebulizer to maintain a constant tidal volume and minute ventilation [4,5]. Obviously, intermittent operation is more efficient for aerosol delivery than continuous aerosol generation [69,70]. When the nebulizer is operated intermittently, the driving pressure provided by some mechanical ventilators may be much lower than that provided by compressed air or oxygen sources. The lower pressure of the driving gas could significantly alter the aerosol characteristics and efficiency of a nebulizer when it is connected in a ventilator circuit. Newer generations of ventilators are being marketed with nebulizers that have been tested to generate aerosols efficiently during intermittent operation [69]. Availability of ventilators with built-in nebulizers will facilitate reproducible and consistent dosing with a variety of agents in ventilated patients [69,71].

The rate of aerosol production is highly variable, not only among various nebulizer brands but even among different batches of the same brand [72–75]. The nature of the aerosol produced, especially particle size, differs among various nebulizer brands [7,74–76]. Furthermore, the operational

Table 4
Problems with CFC-propelled pMDIs, changes made in HFA-propelled pMDIs and their clinical implications

CFC-pMDI	Changes in HFA-pMDI	Clinical implication
Aerosol plume [29,30,52,53,57–59]		
High velocity	Reduced velocity	Decreased oropharyngeal deposition
Cold temperature	Warmer	Reduced chances of "cold-freon" effect
Spray emitted as a jet	Rounder configuration	Difference in feel and taste
Metering Chamber		
Volume 50 μL–100 μL	Smaller chamber	Less chance of leakage during storage
		Lesser chances of loss of prime
Formulation [30,31,34,60]		
Creaming of suspension	Solution, ethanol used as solvent/cosolvent	No need to shake the aerosol before use
Variable puff to puff dosing	Improved puff to puff dosing	More consistent clinical efficacy
Tail-off effect after recommended number of doses	Only few additional doses provided after recommended number of doses	Less chance of misuse because spray content decreases markedly when canister is empty
Actuator nozzle [61–63]		
Nozzle diameter 0.14 mm–0.6 mm	Smaller sized aperture	Greater chances of clogging with potential to change aerosol characteristics; recommended to wash actuator once weekly.
	Finer aerosol particle size	Reduced oropharyngeal deposition. In combination with reduced spray velocity enhances efficiency of drug deposition in the lung
Dose counter [64]		
No dose counter	Dose counter on some	Less chance of under or overdosing as patients can count the number of doses employed and determine when canister is empty
Moisture affinity [35]		
Moisture leaks into canister	Increased moisture affinity	Some HFA-pMDIs (eg, Ventolin) have lower shelf-life after being removed from water-resistant pouch
Temperature dependence [29]		
Operates best in warm temperature	Less temperature dependence	Less chance of losing efficacy in cold weather
Cost [65]		
Generic inhalers inexpensive	Higher cost of name brand pMDIs	Could change cost-benefit of using pMDIs

efficiency of a nebulizer changes with the pressure of the driving gas and with different fill volumes. Moreover, ventilator mode (pressure versus volume controlled ventilation) and lung mechanics could also influence drug delivery from a nebulizer [77]. Before employing a nebulizer in a ventilated patient, it is imperative to characterize its efficiency in a ventilator circuit under the typical clinical conditions in which it will be employed [69].

Placing a jet nebulizer at a distance from the endotracheal tube improves its efficiency, compared with placing it between the patient Y-piece and endotracheal tube [70,78,79]. Addition of a reservoir between the nebulizer and endotracheal tube also modestly increases efficiency of drug delivery [80]. Under these conditions, the aerosol is retained in the reservoir or the inspiratory tubing distal to the nebulizer until it is cleared by the inspiratory airflow. In this way, aerosol wastage during the expiratory phase of the breathing cycle is reduced.

Ultrasonic nebulizers

In ultrasonic nebulizers, aerosol particle size and drug output are influenced by the vibration frequency and amplitude of vibration of the piezo-electric crystal, respectively [81,82]. Thus,

similarly to jet nebulizers, the efficiency of ultrasonic nebulizers depends on the brand of nebulizer
employed. Several brands of ultrasonic nebulizers
that are commercially available have been employed for aerosol delivery during mechanical
ventilation. The SUN 345 (Siemens-Elema AB,
Solna, Sweden) was adapted for use with the
Siemens 300 series of ventilators. Likewise, the
Easy Neb was marketed for use with the Puritan
Bennett 700 and 800 series of ventilators (Puritan
Bennett, Pleasanton, California). The SUN 145
is another ultrasonic nebulizer introduced by
Siemens for continuous use with a variety of ventilators. Most ultrasonic nebulizers have a higher
rate of nebulization and require a shorter time
of operation than jet nebulizers [83].

Ultrasonic nebulizers have not gained popularity for aerosol delivery during mechanical
ventilation because of several problems associated
with their use. Generally, the aerosol particle size
is larger with ultrasonic nebulizers, as compared
to jet nebulizers. Their bulk and relative ineffi-
ciency in nebulizing drug suspensions are other
major limitations to the use of ultrasonic nebulizers. To overcome the problem of size, smaller
volume ultrasonic nebulizers with smaller residual
volumes than jet nebulizers have been employed
[83,84]. The contained portable power source also
makes such ultrasonic nebulizers more easily portable and convenient to use. However, these
devices are much more expensive than jet nebulizers. Another problem with ultrasonic nebulizers
is that the drug solution becomes more concen-
trated during operation, and the solution temperature increases by 10°C to 15°C after a few
minutes of ultrasonic nebulization [85,86]. The
increase in temperature has the potential to
denature some drug formulations.

Placement of ultrasonic nebulizers proximal to
or distal to the Y-piece in the ventilator circuit
does not influence the efficiency of aerosol delivery
[79,87]. Likewise, placing the ultrasonic nebulizer
in the inspiratory limb of the ventilator circuit
50 cm from the Y-piece did not improve its efficiency [87]. The efficiency of aerosol delivery
with ultrasonic nebulizers could be modestly improved by employing a longer inspiratory time,
by reducing the minute ventilation, and by employing a lower respiratory rate [79,87]. Notably,
the efficiency of aerosol delivery with ultrasonic
nebulizers is doubled by the addition of a cylindric
storage chamber (volume 500 mL–600 mL) in
the inspiratory limb of the ventilator circuit
[79,87].

In ventilator-supported patients, ultrasonic
nebulizers are unlikely to gain much popularity
because of their high cost and the other problems
mentioned above. Moreover, newer generation
nebulizers that are specifically designed for in-
line use (see next secion) are now commercially
available and will likely be preferred to traditional
ultrasonic nebulizers for aerosol delivery in ventilator-dependent patients.

Vibrating mesh nebulizers

Newer generations of nebulizers employ a vibrating mesh or plate with multiple apertures to
produce an aerosol [7,68,88–92]. These devices
can be operated either with a battery pack or electrical source, and they are portable and less noisy
than conventional jet nebulizers. Moreover, these
devices have higher drug output because their
residual volume is negligible [7,92]. The Aeroneb
Pro (Aerogen Inc., Mountain View, California)
is specifically designed as an in-line nebulizer;
a breath-synchronized version of the Aeroneb
Pro (Pulmonary Drug Delivery System, PDDS,
Aerogen, Inc) is undergoing clinical trials [7].
The control module of the PDDS is microprocessor driven and uses a pressure transducer to monitor changes in airway pressure and identify
inspiratory time. The microprocessor delivers
aerosol only during a specified portion of the
inspiration. The PDDS generates a fine particle
aerosol that delivers inhaled amikacin with
a high-efficiency (approximately 60% of the nominal dose) in ventilated patients [7].

The vibrating mesh nebulizers have a high rate
of nebulization and drug output is two to three
times higher than with jet nebulizers [7,88]. Unlike
ultrasonic nebulizers, the temperature of the solution does not change during operation of the
vibrating mesh nebulizers, and proteins and pep-
tides can be nebulized with minimal risk of dena-
turation [88,92]. The vibrating mesh nebulizers
have many advantages over jet nebulizers and
they are likely to find increasing use for delivery
of specific (nonbronchodilator) aerosols in ventilator-dependent patients [7,66].

Selection of an aerosol delivery device

Traditionally, pMDIs have been prescribed for
out-patient treatment of airway obstruction,
whereas nebulizers have been widely used during
in-hospital visits. This has led to the erroneous
belief that nebulizers are preferred for bronchodilator delivery in critically ill patients. Bronchodilator therapy with either pMDIs or nebulizers

produces similar therapeutic effects in ventilator-supported patients [4,6,16,18]. In fact, when employed in an optimal manner, pMDIs and nebulizers are equally effective in the treatment of mechanically ventilated patients with obstructive lung disease [93]. For routine bronchodilator therapy, pMDIs are preferred because of their convenience, more consistent dosing, and reduced chances of bacterial contamination [94,95]. In one survey of neonatal ICUs, pMDI use was reported to have increased significantly over a period of approximately 10 years [96]. Although there has been no formal survey, the majority of adult ICUs in the United States also prefer pMDIs for routine bronchodilator therapy [97]. Nebulizers continue to be employed for a proportion of bronchodilator treatments, and for delivery of antibiotics, surfactant, prostaglandins, and other formulations that are not available in pMDIs [4,66]. Previously bronchodilator administration with pMDIs was thought to be more cost effective than nebulizers [98–100]; however, this may no longer hold true as we transition from the generic CFC-pMDIs to the branded HFA-pMDIs.

Aerosol particle size

During mechanical ventilation, larger particles produced by pMDIs and nebulizers are trapped in the ventilator circuit and endotracheal tube (Fig. 4); therefore, devices that produce aerosols with MMAD less than 2 μm are more efficient during mechanical ventilation than devices that produce aerosols with larger particles [51,101–103]. Nebulizers and pMDIs delivered an equivalent mass of aerosol beyond the endotracheal tube in a ventilator model [48]. While nebulizers that produce aerosols with smaller particle sizes have been employed during mechanical ventilation, they require a considerably greater time to deliver a standard dose [69,101]. The aerosol particle size with vibrating mesh nebulizers is variable [7,91], but a significant proportion of the aerosol generated is in particles less than 3.3 μm in size (the fine particle fraction) [90,91].

Conditions in the ventilator circuit

Humidity

The gas in the ventilator circuit is heated and humidified to prevent drying of the airway mucosa. Humidification leads to an increased loss of aerosol in the ventilator circuit [51] and reduces

drug delivery to the lower respiratory tract from both MDIs and nebulizers by 40% or more in a humidified, as compared with a dry, circuit (Fig. 5) [4,5,69,104]. Although circuit humidity reduces drug delivery, bypassing the humidifier is not recommended for routine inhalation therapy in ventilator-supported patients. With careful attention to the technique of administration, the impact of humidity on drug delivery can be overcome by delivering a somewhat higher drug dose [11,12,14,18]. A dry circuit could be employed for delivery of those agents that are very expensive or those agents for which the amount of drug deposition is critical (eg, antibiotics and prostaglandins). When a dry circuit is employed, drug administration should be achieved within a short period (less than 10 to 15 minutes) to minimize the effects of dry gas on the airway mucosa.

Heat and moisture exchangers (HMEs) are passive humidification systems that capture the heat and moisture from the exhaled breath and transfer part of the heat and humidity to the next inspired breath [105]. HMEs are often employed to provide humidification of inspired air during mechanical ventilation [105]. The filter in the HME is a barrier to aerosol delivery and the device must be removed from the circuit during aerosol delivery. The Circuvent (DHD Health Care Corp. Wampsville, New York) allows aerosol delivery without removing the HME from the circuit. A piece of tubing bypasses the HME and this circuit is employed during aerosol generation by turning a dial on the device. After aerosol generation is completed, the dial is turned back to allow inspiratory airflow to pass through the HME. The efficiency of aerosol delivery by this device has not been established in clinical studies.

Gas density

Inhalation of a less dense gas than air or oxygen, such as helium-oxygen 70/30 mixture, improves drug delivery in both pediatric and adult models of mechanical ventilation [106,107]. Likewise, studies in ambulatory patients have shown higher aerosol retention in the lungs when patients breathed heliox instead of air [108,109]. Helium-oxygen could be employed to increase aerosol delivery to the lung. With pMDIs there may be as much as a 50% increase in the amount of aerosol delivered to the lower respiratory tract when helium-oxygen is employed, compared with air or oxygen (Fig. 6) [107]. In contrast, nebulizer

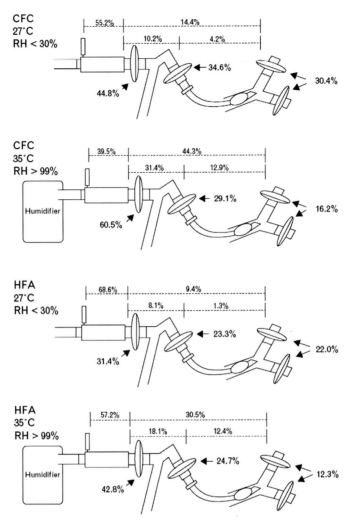

Fig. 4. Drug deposition, expressed as percent of nominal dose of albuterol from a CFC-propelled pMDI, in the spacer chamber, the ventilator circuit, the endotracheal tube, and on filters at the bronchi under dry and humidified conditions during controlled mechanical ventilation. Under dry conditions, 30.4% of the dose from a CFC-pMDI was deposited at the bronchi. The presence of humidity in the circuit reduced the delivery at the same site to 16.2%. With an albuterol HFA-propelled pMDI under dry conditions, 22.0% of the drug was delivered at the bronchi. The presence of humidity in the circuit reduced the delivery at the same site to 12.3%. Under both dry and humidified conditions drug delivery to the bronchi with the albuterol HFA-propelled pMDI was lower than that with the CFC-propelled pMDI. RH = relative humidity. (*From* Fink JB, Dhand R, Grychowski J, et al. Reconciling in-vitro and in-vivo measurements of aerosol delivery from a metered-dose inhaler during mechanical ventilation, and defining efficiency enhancing factors. Am J Respir Crit Care Med 1999;159:63–8; with permission.)

operation with helium-oxygen reduced drug output and respirable mass (see Fig. 6) [107,110]. A practical method to achieve maximum pulmonary deposition of aerosol from a nebulizer during mechanical ventilation is to operate the nebulizer with oxygen at a flow rate of 6 L to 8 L per minute and to entrain the aerosol generated into a ventilator circuit containing helium-oxygen [107].

Artificial airway

Aerosol impaction on the endotracheal tube poses a significant barrier to effective drug delivery in infant and pediatric mechanical ventilation (endotracheal tube internal diameter of 3 mm–6 mm) [102,111]. In adult mechanical ventilation, there was no difference in nebulizer

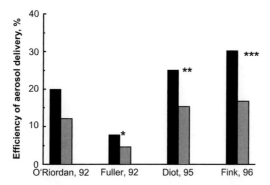

Fig. 5. Effect of humidity on aerosol delivery. The delivery of aerosol to the lower respiratory tract in bench models of mechanical ventilation is reduced by approximately 40% when the circuit is humidified versus dry. *, $P<.05$; **, $P<.01$; ***, $P<.001$. Black bars = Dry. Gray bars = Humid. Studies: O'Riordan et al [101], Fuller et al [49], Diot et al [48], Fink et al [113]. (*From* Dhand R, Tobin MJ. Inhaled bronchodilator therapy in mechanically ventilated patients. Am J Respir Crit Care Med 1997;156:3–10; with permission.)

efficiency with endotracheal tubes of internal diameter 7 mm versus an internal diameter of 9 mm [78]. Drug losses within the endotracheal tube could be minimized by placing the aerosol generator at a distance from the endotracheal tube instead of being directly connected to it [112]. When a pMDI and spacer are employed, the presence of humidity in the circuit increased aerosol deposition in the endotracheal tube by approximately threefold (see Fig. 4) [4,51,113]. In vitro studies show minimal drug deposition

within endotracheal tubes with jet nebulizers; however, significant endotracheal tube deposition of aerosol occurs with ultrasonic nebulizers [83].

Aerosol deposition in tracheostomy tubes has not been studied in as much detail as endotracheal tubes. By using a mass balance technique, O'Riordan and colleagues [101] found that approximately 10% of the nominal dose from a nebulizer deposited in the tracheostomy tube of mechanically ventilated patients. The majority of aerosol deposition (approximately 7%)

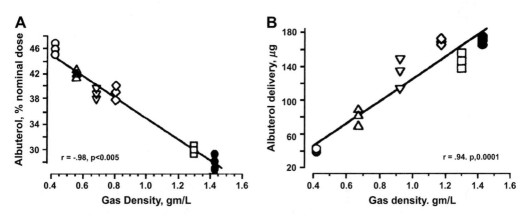

Fig. 6. Effect of gas density on aerosol delivery from an MDI and jet nebulizer. In panel *A*, albuterol was administered via an MDI and chamber spacer in an unheated dry ventilator circuit containing air (*squares*), 100% oxygen (*black circles*), or several mixtures of helium-oxygen: 80/20 (*white circles*), 70/30 (*triangles*), 60/40 (*inverted triangles*), and 50/50 (*diamonds*). Albuterol delivery from a MDI (percent of nominal dose) was inversely related ($r = -0.98$; $P<.005$) to gas density. In panel *B*, albuterol was administered with a jet nebulizer operated at a constant flow of 6 L per minute of air (*squares*), 100% oxygen (*black circles*), or helium-oxygen mixtures—80/20 (*white circles*), 60/40 (*triangles*), 40/60 (*inverted triangles*), 20/80 (*diamonds*)—and albuterol output from the nebulizer was measured. Albuterol output from the nebulizer was positively correlated ($r = 0.94$; $P<.0001$) with the density of gas used to operate the nebulizer. (*Adapted from* Goode ML, Fink JB, Dhand R, et al. Improvement in aerosol delivery with helium-oxygen mixtures during mechanical ventilation. Am J Respir Crit Care Med 2001;163:109–14; with permission.)

occurred during exhalation. Because in vitro studies are unable to directly determine aerosol deposition during exhalation, such studies could significantly underestimate the actual deposition of aerosol in the artificial airway.

Ventilatory parameters

Synchronizing aerosol generation with inspiratory airflow

The actuation of a MDI must be synchronized with the precise onset of inspiratory airflow from the ventilator [4,48,114]. As short as a 1- to 1.5-second delay between MDI actuation and a ventilator breath can profoundly reduce the efficiency of drug delivery [48]. Likewise, intermittent operation of the nebulizer that is synchronized with inspiratory airflow from the ventilator is more efficient for aerosol delivery, compared with continuous aerosol generation, because it minimizes aerosol wastage during the exhalation phase of the breathing cycle [69,70]. The lower driving pressure provided by the ventilator (less than 15 psi) than that provided by pressurized gas (greater than or equal to 50 psi) could decrease the efficiency of some nebulizers [115]. Aerosol generated by a nebulizer operating at the lower pressure may generate particles whose diameter is larger than the 1 μm to 5 μm that is considered to be optimal for aerosol delivery. When intermittent nebulizer operation is employed, the specific ventilator and nebulizer brand should be tested to determine the characteristics of the aerosol generated and the efficiency of drug delivery [69,71].

Characteristics of the ventilator breath

The characteristics of the ventilator breath have an important influence on aerosol drug delivery. A tidal volume of 500 mL or more (in an adult) [113], longer inspiratory time, and slower inspiratory flows improve aerosol delivery [113,116,117]. Drug delivery is linearly correlated with a longer duty cycle (T_I/T_{TOT}): that is, the ratio of the inspiratory time (T_I) to the total duration of the breathing cycle (T_{TOT}), for both pMDIs and nebulizers [51,78,113,117]. Moreover, drug delivery is improved when a pMDI is synchronized with a simulated spontaneous breath, compared with a controlled ventilator breath of similar tidal volume [113]. However, altering ventilatory parameters does not influence bronchodilator response to albuterol in mechanically ventilated patients with COPD [14,15,17].

The inspiratory waveform influences drug delivery from nebulizers but has much less influence on drug delivery from a pMDI [77]. Unlike pMDIs, nebulizer efficiency is notably lower during pressure-controlled ventilation than during volume-controlled ventilation [77]. The breath-triggering mechanism does not significantly influence drug delivery from a pMDI, but use of a flow trigger with a nebulizer could dilute the aerosol and increase the washout of the aerosol into the expiratory limb between breaths [113].

In mechanically-ventilated patients with COPD, the application of external positive end-expiratory pressure (PEEP) at a level that counterbalanced intrinsic PEEP enhanced the bronchodilator effect of albuterol and improved gas exchange and hemodynamics [19]. The additive effects of external PEEP and albuterol may be explained by the effect of albuterol in reducing time-constant inequality, thereby producing alveolar recruitment during tidal ventilation, and the application of external PEEP could maintain this alveolar recruitment. Thus, external PEEP could enhance aerosol drug deposition in the peripheral airways.

Tzoufi and colleagues [19] observed that the level of intrinsic PEEP was markedly reduced by the combination of albuterol and external PEEP. In contrast, Guerin and colleagues [118] did not observe an additional effect on respiratory mechanics in mechanically ventilated subjects with COPD when nebulized fenoterol was administered with external PEEP set at 80% of total PEEP, compared with the same drug administered with external PEEP set at zero. The discrepancy between the results of the two studies may be related to the fact that Tzoufi and colleagues measured the responses 30 minutes after albuterol, whereas Guerin and coworkers measured the responses to fenoterol for up to 240 minutes. The effect of bronchodilators to reduce intrinsic PEEP may be initially beneficial; however, with the passage of time the levels of intrinsic PEEP may fall below the set external PEEP. Application of external PEEP could then be counterproductive. Thus, in patients receiving bronchodilators, the external PEEP levels would need to be periodically monitored to ensure that they are not higher than the levels of intrinsic PEEP.

Efficiency of drug delivery during mechanical ventilation

In the past, pMDIs and nebulizers were shown to have poor efficiency for aerosol delivery during mechanical ventilation [1,2]. MacIntyre and colleagues [1] did not observe a bronchodilator response in 15 mechanically ventilated subjects who received inhaled metaproterenol sulfate by jet nebulizer attached to the proximal end of the endotracheal tube. Subsequently, bench studies with simulated models of mechanical ventilation [4,9,47,48,50,51,55,56,69,70,77–79,87,101,102,105, 106,111,113,115], scintigraphy with radio-labeled aerosols [1,2,83,87,101], and pharmacokinetic studies [119,120] in subjects have been employed to optimize techniques of administration with various aerosol generators. With a standardized technique of administration, approximately 11% of the nominal dose from a pMDI and spacer chamber deposits in the lower respiratory tract of ventilated patients [51]. This value is remarkably close to values observed (10%–14%) with the optimal use of a pMDI without a spacer in ambulatory patients [121,122].

Drug delivery from nebulizers also shows discrepancy between values obtained with bench models versus those obtained by gamma scintigraphy. Miller and colleagues [69] found that accounting for circuit humidity and breath-actuated nebulization could reconcile most observed differences. With an optimal technique of administration, an estimated 6% to 10% of the nominal dose placed in the nebulizer would be inhaled by a patient breathing through a humidified ventilator circuit [69]. A significant proportion of the inhaled mass deposits in the endotracheal tube and a smaller proportion is exhaled. Thus, the efficiency of drug deposition in the lower respiratory tract of ventilated patients is lower with nebulizers than with pMDIs. Higher drug doses are employed with nebulizers to offset their reduced efficiency [18]. The total amount of drug depositing in the lower respiratory tract with jet nebulizers is probably comparable to that achieved with smaller drug doses employed with a pMDI.

Vecellio and colleagues [123] demonstrated that the amount of drug delivered to the lung with a nebulizer could be estimated under specified conditions of nebulizer operation. These investigators determined the factors influencing drug delivery from a nebulizer in a bench model of mechanical ventilation. Once the drug output per minute was known, the time required to deliver a predetermined quantity of drug under the specified ventilatory conditions could be estimated.

In summary, many investigators using different techniques of evaluation have studied aerosol delivery during mechanical ventilation. These studies have established the scientific basis of aerosol therapy in mechanically ventilated patients and helped to formulate the optimal techniques of aerosol administration in this patient population.

Technique of administration

Variations in the efficiency of pMDIs and nebulizers to deliver aerosol to the lung in mechanically ventilated patients underscore the need for carefully controlling the technique of administration. The recommended techniques of administration with pMDIs and nebulizers are shown in Boxes 2 and 3 [124], respectively. With pMDIs the key steps are to employ an in-line chamber spacer and to synchronize the actuation of the pMDI with onset of inspiratory airflow from the ventilator [4,23,51,113]. With nebulizers, a device that produces an aerosol with the majority of drug contained in particles smaller than 3 μm is ideal. Intermittent operation of the nebulizer and placement at a distance from the patient also enhance drug deposition in the lung [4,66,69].

Inhalation therapy and clinical outcomes

Inhaled bronchodilators are frequently employed in ventilator-supported patients [125]. However, the effects of bronchodilator therapy on clinically relevant outcomes, such as the duration of mechanical ventilation, length of ICU stay, length of hospital stay, in-hospital mortality, or long-term mortality, are not known. In patients with airflow obstruction, inhaled bronchodilators improve wheezing [126], hemodynamics [19], reduce airway resistance, and intrinsic PEEP levels [11,12,19,118]. Improvement in lung mechanics has been noted even among patients with no known airflow obstruction [127–129]. Bronchodilators also reduce the work of breathing [130], and they could reduce the sensation of dyspnea while improving patient-ventilator interaction. Bronchodilators could facilitate weaning in patients with limited cardiopulmonary reserve [130]. In addition, they may improve mucociliary clearance [131] and facilitate clearance of pulmonary edema [132]. Combining beta-2 adrenergic and anticholinergic bronchodilators has a greater effect than therapy with either agent alone [133]. However, higher doses of beta-agonists have the potential to cause hypokalemia and cardiac arrhythmias [8,134–136]. Unfortunately, no randomized controlled trials have been performed to evaluate the effect of bronchodilator therapy

---

Box 2. Optimal technique for drug delivery by pMDI in ventilated patients

Review order, identify patient, and assess need for bronchodilator.
Suction endotracheal tube and airway secretions.
Shake pMDI and warm to hand temperature.
Place pMDI in space chamber adapter in ventilator circuit.
Remove HME. Do not disconnect humidifier.
Coordinate pMDI actuation with beginning of inspiration.
Wait at least 15 seconds between actuations; administer total dose.
Monitor for adverse response.
Reconnect HME.
Document clinical outcome.

---

on clinically relevant outcomes in ventilator-supported patients [93,97,137]. Moreover, variations in the method of administration and assessment of response make it difficult to compare the results of various studies [93].

The role of bronchodilators in mechanically ventilated patients without airflow obstruction is even less obvious. Chang and colleagues [97] found no difference in incidence of ventilator-associated pneumonia or mortality among ventilator-supported patients without obstructive lung disease. There was a trend toward longer duration of mechanical ventilation in patients receiving bronchodilator therapy. However, this could be explained by a bias for bronchodilator therapy in patients who had pneumonia and lower arterial oxygen tension more frequently than those not receiving such therapy. In general, clinical outcomes did not improve with bronchodilator therapy [97]. At the same time, bronchodilator treatment was safe and was associated with a modest increase in the cost of treatment [97].

Further studies are needed to evaluate the influence of inhaled bronchodilators on clinically relevant outcomes in ventilator-dependent patients. Likewise, the role of other inhaled therapies, such as surfactant, antibiotics, prostaglandins, mucolytics, and other inhalents, also need to be established by randomized, controlled trials in ventilator-supported patients.

Box 3. Optimal technique for drug delivery by jet nebulizer in ventilated patients

Review order, identify patient, and assess need for bronchodilator.
Suction endotracheal and airway secretions.
Place drug in nebulizer to fill volume of 4 mL to 6 mL.
Place nebulizer in the inspiratory line 18 inches (46 cm) from the patient y-piece.
Turn off flow-by or continuous flow during nebulizer operation.
Remove HME from circuit (do not disconnect humidifier).
Set gas flow to nebulizer at 6 L to 8 L per minute.
  Use a ventilator if it meets the nebulizer flow requirements and cycles on inspiration, or
  Use continuous flow from external source.
Adjust ventilator volume or pressure limit to compensate for added flow.
Tap nebulizer periodically until nebulizer begins to sputter.
Remove nebulizer from circuit, rinse with sterile water and run dry, store in safe place.
Reconnect humidifier or HME, return ventilator settings and alarms to previous values.
Monitor patient for adverse response.
Assess outcome and document findings.

Data from Fink J. Aerosol drug therapy. In: Wilkins RL, Stoller JK, Scanlan CL, editors. Egan's fundamentals of respiratory care. 8th edition. St. Louis (MO): Mosby; 2003. p. 761–800.

Aerosol delivery during noninvasive positive pressure ventilation

Noninvasive positive-pressure ventilation (NPPV) is being increasingly employed for treatment of patients with acute and chronic respiratory failure [138]. NPPV may be employed as a first line mode of mechanical ventilation in as many as 50% of patients with hypercapnic respiratory failure [138]. Successful application of NPPV with a nasal or facemask can often obviate the need for endotracheal intubation and improve mortality [139–143]. Inhaled bronchodilators are often administered to patients with acute or acute-on-chronic hypercapnic respiratory failure who are receiving NPPV. In the past, acutely ill patients routinely received bronchodilators with intermittent positive-pressure breathing devices [144,145], until it was determined that drug delivery was reduced by this technique of administration [146]. However, there may be a role for employing positive pressure ventilation in acutely ill patients requiring ventilatory support, as conventional methods of administering pMDIs or nebulizers may not provide optimal aerosol delivery in this setting [147].

The optimal techniques for aerosol delivery in patients receiving NPPV have been investigated with in vitro models. Similarly to invasive positive pressure ventilation, aerosol delivery can vary as much as fivefold (5% versus 25% of the nominal dose) during NPPV, depending on the inspiratory and expiratory pressures employed, position of the nebulizer, and synchronization of pMDI actuation with inhalation [148–150].

Although the optimum settings required for maximum drug delivery with a pMDI during NPPV have not been established, significant bronchodilator responses occur after albuterol administration with a jet nebulizer or a pMDI in stable patients [145,151], and in patients with acute asthma exacerbations receiving NPPV with mask [152]. Similarly to invasive mechanical ventilation, the use of helium-oxygen mixtures has beneficial effects in patients with COPD receiving NPPV [153]. Both pMDIs and nebulizers could be employed, but further studies are needed to optimize drug delivery from these devices during NPPV.

Summary

Delivery of aerosols to patients receiving mechanical ventilation is complex; many factors influence the amount of drug deposition in the lower respiratory tract, and the technique of administration needs to be carefully controlled. Optimal techniques for employing pMDIs and nebulizers have been developed as a result of better understanding of the factors influencing aerosol delivery to the lower respiratory tract of ventilator-dependent patients. With a proper technique of administration, drug deposition in the lower respiratory tract of ventilator-supported patients is comparable to that achieved in ambulatory patients. For routine therapy, a somewhat higher dose than that employed in ambulatory patients is recommended in mechanically ventilated patients to compensate for the effects of humidity in the ventilator circuit. Currently, there is increasing emphasis on the use of NPPV as first-line therapy for patients requiring ventilator support, but only a few investigators have studied aerosol delivery in this setting. Growing understanding of the factors influencing delivery of aerosols during mechanical ventilation, coupled with the availability of highly efficient delivery devices, is leading to increasing application of inhaled therapies in ventilated patients.

Acknowledgment

The authors thank Lauren Elliott for her help and support in the preparation of this manuscript.

References

[1] MacIntyre NR, Silver RM, Miller CW, et al. Aerosol delivery in intubated, mechanically ventilated patients. Crit Care Med 1985;13:81–4.

[2] Fuller HD, Dolovich MB, Posmituck G, et al. Pressurized aerosol versus jet aerosol delivery to mechanically ventilated patients. Comparison of dose to the lungs. Am Rev Respir Dis 1990;141:440–4.

[3] Aerosol consensus statement–1991. American Association for Respiratory Care. Respir Care 1991;36(9):916–21.

[4] Dhand R. Bronchodilator therapy. In: Tobin M, editor. Principles and practice of mechanical ventilation. 2nd edition. New York: McGraw Hill; 2006. p. 1277–310.

[5] Dhand R, Tobin MJ. Inhaled drug therapy in mechanically-ventilated patients. (Pulmonary Perspective). Am J Respir Crit Care Med 1997; 156:3–10.

[6] Dhand R. Inhalation therapy with metered-dose inhalers and dry powder inhalers in mechanically-ventilated patients. Respir Care 2005;50(10): 1331–44 [discussion: 1344–45].

[7] Dhand R, Sohal H. Pulmonary Drug Delivery System for inhalation therapy in mechanically ventilated patients. Expert Rev Med Devices 2008;5(1):9–18.

[8] Manthous CA, Hall JB, Schmidt GA, et al. Metered-dose inhaler versus nebulized albuterol in mechanically ventilated patients. Am Rev Respir Dis 1993;148:1567–70.

[9] Rau JL, Harwood RJ, Groff JL. Evaluation of a reservoir device for metered-dose bronchodilator delivery to intubated adults: an in vitro study. Chest 1992;102:924–30.

[10] Manthous CA, Chatila W, Schmidt GA, et al. Treatment of bronchospasm by metered-dose inhaler albuterol in mechanically ventilated patients. Chest 1995;107:210–3.

[11] Dhand R, Jubran A, Tobin MJ. Bronchodilator delivery by metered-dose inhaler in ventilator-supported patients. Am J Respir Crit Care Med. 1995;151(6):1827–33.

[12] Dhand R, Duarte AG, Jubran A, et al. Dose-response to bronchodilator delivered by metered-dose inhaler in ventilator-supported patients. Am J Respir Crit Care Med 1996;154:388–93.

[13] Waugh JB, Jones DF, Aranson R, et al. Bronchodilator response with use of OptiVent versus Aerosol Cloud Enhancer metered-dose inhaler spacers in patients receiving ventilatory assistance. Heart Lung 1998;27:418–23.

[14] Mouloudi E, Katsanoulas K, Anastasaki M, et al. Bronchodilator delivery by metered-dose inhaler in mechanically ventilated COPD patients: influence of end-inspiratory pause. Eur Respir J 1998;12:165–9.

[15] Mouloudi E, Katsanoulas K, Anastasaki M, et al. Bronchodilator delivery by metered-dose inhaler in mechanically ventilated COPD patients: influence of tidal volume. Intensive Care Med 1999;25:1215–21.

[16] Guerin C, Chevre A, Dessirier P, et al. Inhaled fenoterol-ipratropium bromide in mechanically ventilated patients with chronic obstructive pulmonary disease. Am J Respir Crit Care Med 1999;159: 1036–42.

[17] Mouloudi E, Prinianakis G, Kondili E, et al. Bronchodilator delivery by metered-dose inhaler in mechanically ventilated COPD patients: influence of flow pattern. Eur Respir J 2000;16: 263–8.

[18] Duarte AG, Momii K, Bidani A. Bronchodilator therapy with metered-dose inhaler and spacer versus nebulizer in mechanically ventilated patients: comparison of magnitude and duration of response. Respir Care 2000;45(7):817–23.

[19] Tzoufi M, Mentzelopoulos SD, Roussos C, et al. The effects of nebulized salbutamol, external positive end-expiratory pressure, and their combination on respiratory mechanics, hemodynamics, and gas exchange in mechanically ventilated chronic obstructive pulmonary disease patients. Anesth Analg 2005;101(3):843–50.

[20] Dhand R. Aerosol delivery during mechanical ventilation: from basic techniques to new devices. J Aerosol Med 2008;21:45–60.

[21] Gay PC, Patel HG, Nelson SB, et al. Metered dose inhalers for bronchodilator delivery in intubated, mechanically ventilated patients. Chest 1991;99: 66–71.

[22] Bates JH, Milic-Emili J. The flow interruption technique for measuring respiratory resistance. J Crit Care 1991;6:227–38.

[23] Dhand R. Bronchodilator delivery with metered-dose inhalers in mechanically ventilated patients. Eur Respir J 1996;9:585–95.

[24] Hendeles L, Colice GL, Meyer RJ. Withdrawal of albuterol inhalers containing chlorofluorocarbon propellants. N Engl J Med 2007;356:1344–51.

[25] Food and Drug Administration. Use of ozone-depleting substances: removal of essential-use designation. Final rule. Fed Regist 2005;70: 17167–92.

[26] Moren F. Aerosol dosage forms and formulations. In: Moren F, Dolovich MB, Newhouse MT, et al, editors. Aerosols in medicine: principles, diagnosis and therapy. 2nd edition. Amsterdam: Elsevier; 1993. p. 321–50.

[27] Dockhorn R, Vanden Burgt JA, Ekholm BP, et al. Clinical equivalence of a novel non-chlorofluorocarbon containing salbutamol sulfate metered-dose inhaler and a conventional chloro-fluorocarbon inhaler in patients with asthma. J Allergy Clin Immunol 1995;96:50–6.

[28] Vervaet C, Byron PR. Drug-surfactant-propellant interactions in HFA formulations. Int J Pharm 1999;186(1):13–20.

[29] Leach C. Enhanced drug delivery through reformulating MDIs with HFA propellants—drug deposition and its effect on preclinical and clinical programs. Respiratory Drug Delivery V. Buffalo Grove (IL): Interpharm Press Inc.; 1996. p. 133–44.

[30] Ross DL, Gabrio BJ. Advances in metered-dose inhaler technology with the development of a chlorofluorocarbon-free drug delivery system. J Aerosol Med 1999;12:151–60.

[31] Lewis DA, Ganderton D, Meakin BJ, et al. Theory and practice with solution systems. In: Dalby RN, Byron PR, Peart J, et al, editors. Respiratory drug delivery IX. River Grove (IL): Davis Healthcare International; 2004. p. 109–15.

[32] Leach CL, Davidson PJ, Boudreau RJ. Improved airway targeting with the CFC-free HFA-beclomethasone metered-dose inhaler compared with the CFC-beclomethasone. Eur Respir J 1998;12:1346–53.

[33] Gross G, Thompson PJ, Chervinsky P, et al. Hydrofluoroalkane-134a beclomethasone dipropionate, 400 microg, is as effective as chlorofluorocarbon beclomethasone dipropionate, 800 microg,

for the treatment of moderate asthma. Chest 1999; 115:343–51.

[34] Schultz RK. Drug delivery characteristics of metered-dose inhalers. J Allergy Clin Immunol 1995;96:284–7.

[35] Williams G. Moisture transport into chlofluorocarbon-free metered-dose inhalers. J Allergy Clin Immunol 1999;104:S227–9.

[36] Bleecker ER, Tinkelman DG, Ramsdell J, et al. Proventil HFA provides bronchodilation comparable to ventolin over 12 weeks of regular use in asthmatics. Chest 1998;113:283–9.

[37] Shapiro GS, Klinger NM, Ekholm BP, et al. Comparable bronchodilation with hydrofluoroalkane-134a (HFA) albuterol and chlorofluorcarbons-11/12 (CFC) albuterol in children with asthma. J Asthma 2000;37:667–75.

[38] Bronsky E, Ekholm BP, Klinger NM, et al. Switching patients with asthma from chlorofluorocarbon (CFC) albuterol to hydrofluoroalkane-134a (HFA) albuterol. J Asthma 1999;36:107–14.

[39] Lumry W, Noveck R, Weinstein S, et al. Switching from ventolin CFC to ventolin HFA is well tolerated and effective in patients with asthma. Ann Allergy Asthma Immunol 2001;86:297–303.

[40] Parameswaran K, Inman MD, Ekholm BP, et al. Protection against methacholine bronchoconstriction to assess relative potency of inhaled β2-agonist. Am J Respir Crit Care Med 1999;160: 354–7.

[41] Salat D, Popov D, Sykes AP. Equivalence of salbutamol 200 µg four times daily propelled by propellants 11 and 12 or HFA 134a in mild to moderate asthmatics. Respir Med 2000;94:S22–8.

[42] Baumgarten CR, Dorow P, Weber HH, et al. Equivalence of as-required salbutamol propelled by propellants 11 and 12 or HFA 134a in mild to moderate asthmatics. Respir Med 2000;94:S17–21.

[43] Ayres JG, Frost CD, Holmes WF, et al. Postmarketing surveillance study of a non-chlorofluorocarbon inhaler according to the safety assessment of marketed medicines guidelines. BMJ 1998;317:926–30.

[44] Craig-McFeely PM, Wilton LV, Soriano JB, et al. Prospective observational cohort safety study to monitor the introduction of a non-CFC formulation of salbutamol with HFA 134a in England. Int J Clin Pharmacol Ther 2003;41:67–76.

[45] Harrison LI, Cline A, Wells TM, et al. Systemic concentrations of salbutamol and HFA-134a after inhalation of salbutamol sulfate in a chlorofluorocarbon-free system. Ther Drug Monit 1996;18: 240–4.

[46] Rubin BK, Fink JB. Optimizing aerosol delivery by pressurized metered-dose inhalers. Respir Care 2005;50:1191–7.

[47] Bishop MJ, Larson RP, Buschman DL. Metered dose inhaler aerosol characteristics are affected by the endotracheal tube actuator/adapter used. Anesthesiology 1990;73:1263–5.

[48] Diot P, Morra L, Smaldone GC. Albuterol delivery in a model of mechanical ventilation. Comparison of metered-dose inhaler and nebulizer efficiency. Am J Respir Crit Care Med 1995;152:1391–4.

[49] Fuller HD, Dolovich MB, Turpie FH, et al. Efficiency of bronchodilator aerosol delivery to the lungs from the metered dose inhaler in mechanically ventilated patients. A study comparing four different actuator devices. Chest 1994;105: 214–8.

[50] Rau JL, Dunlevy CL, Hill RL. A comparison of inline MDI actuators for delivery of a beta agonist and a corticosteroid with a mechanically-ventilated lung model. Respir Care 1998;43:705–12.

[51] Fink JB, Dhand R, Grychowski J, et al. Reconciling in-vitro and in-vivo measurements of aerosol delivery from a metered-dose inhaler during mechanical ventilation, and defining efficiency enhancing factors. Am J Respir Crit Care Med 1999;159:63–8.

[52] Barry PW, O'Callaghan C. In vitro comparison of the amount of salbutamol available for inhalation from different formulations with different spacer devices. Eur Respir J 1997;10:1345–8.

[53] Gabrio BJ, Stein SW, Velasquez DJ. A new method to evaluate plume characteristics of hydrofluoroalkane and chlorofluorocarbon metered dose inhalers. Int J Pharm 1999;186:3–12.

[54] Mitchell JP, Nagel MW, Wiersema KJ, et al. The delivery of chlorofluorocarbon-propelled versus hydrofluoroalkane-propelled beclomethasone dipropionate aerosol to the mechanically-ventilated patient: a laboratory study. Respir Care 2003;48: 1025–32.

[55] Wildhaber JH, Hayden MJ, Dore ND, et al. Salbutamol delivery from a hydrofluoroalkane pressurized metered-dose inhaler in pediatric ventilator circuits. Chest 1998;113:186–91.

[56] Lugo RA, Kenney JK, Keenan J, et al. Albuterol delivery in a naeonatal ventilated lung model. Pediatr Pulmonol 2001;31:247–54.

[57] Newman S, Pitcairn G, Steed K, et al. Deposition of fenoterol from metered-dose inhalers containing hydrofluoroalkanes. J Allergy Clin Immunol 1999; 104(6):S253–7.

[58] Crompton GK. Problems patients have using pressurized aerosol inhalers. Eur J Respir Dis 1982;63(Suppl 119):57–65.

[59] Brown BAS. Dispelling the myths of MDIs. Drug Delivery technology 2002;2(7):1–7.

[60] Cyr TD, Graham SJ, Li KY, et al. Low first-spray drug content in albuterol metered-dose inhalers. Pharm Res 1991;8:658–60.

[61] Clark AR. MDIs: physics of aerosol formation. J Aerosol Med 1996;9(Suppl 1):S19–26.

[62] Versteeg HK, Hargrave GK, Wigley G. The physics of aerosol formulation by pMDI: an update. Proceedings of Drug Delivery to the Lungs XIII. Portishead: The Aerosol Society;2002;60–66.

[63] Bamber MG. Difficulties with CFC-free salbutamol inhaler. Lancet 1996;348:1737.

[64] Rubin BK, Dorotype L. How do patients determine that their metered-dose inhaler is empty? Chest 2004;126:1134–7.

[65] Food and Drug administration. Use of ozone-depleting substances: removal of essential use designations. Fed Regist 2004;69(115):33602–18.

[66] Dhand R. Inhalation therapy in invasive and noninvasive mechanical ventilation. Curr Opin Crit Care 2007;13(1):27–38.

[67] Dhand R. The role of aerosolized antimicrobials in the treatment of ventilator-associated pneumonia. Respir Care 2007;52(7):866–84.

[68] Diot P, Magro P, Vecellio L, et al. Advances in our understanding of aerosolized iloprost for pulmonary hypertension. J Aerosol Med 2006;19(3):406–7.

[69] Miller DD, Amin MM, Palmer LB, et al. Aerosol delivery and modern mechanical ventilation: in vitro/in vivo evaluation. Am J Respir Crit Care Med 2003;168:1205–9.

[70] Hughes JM, Saez J. Effects of nebulizer mode and position in a mechanical ventilator circuit on dose efficiency. Respir Care 1987;32:1131–5.

[71] Dhand R. Aerosol therapy during mechanical ventilation: getting ready for prime time. Am J Respir Crit Care Med 2003;168(10):1148–9.

[72] Alvine GF, Rodgers P, Fitzsimmons KM, et al. Disposable jet nebulizers. How reliable are they? Chest 1992;101(2):316–9.

[73] Loffert DT, Ikle D, Nelson HS. A comparison of commercial jet nebulizers. Chest 1994;106(6):1788–92.

[74] Waldrep JC, Keyhani K, Black M, et al. Operating characteristics of 18 different continuous-flow jet nebulizers with beclomethasone dipropionate liposome aerosol. Chest 1994;105(1):106–10.

[75] Hess D, Fisher D, Williams P, et al. Medication nebulizer performance. Effects of diluent volume, nebulizer flow, and nebulizer brand. Chest 1996;110(2):498–505.

[76] Sterk PJ, Plomp A, van de Vate JF, et al. Physical properties of aerosols produced by several jet- and ultrasonic nebulizers. Bull Eur Physiopathol Respir 1984;20(1):65–72.

[77] Hess DR, Dillman C, Kacmarek RM. In vitro evaluation of aerosol bronchodilator delivery during mechanical ventilation: pressure-control vs. volume control ventilation. Intensive Care Med 2003;29(7):1145–50.

[78] O'Riordan TG, Greco MJ, Perry RJ, et al. Nebulizer function during mechanical ventilation. Am Rev Respir Dis 1992;145(5):1117–22.

[79] O'Doherty MJ, Thomas SH, Page CJ, et al. Delivery of a nebulized aerosol to a lung model during mechanical ventilation. Effect of ventilator settings and nebulizer type, position, and volume of fill. Am Rev Respir Dis 1992;146:383–8.

[80] Harvey CJ, O'Doherty MJ, Page CJ, et al. Effect of a spacer on pulmonary aerosol deposition from a jet nebuliser during mechanical ventilation. Thorax 1995;50(1):50–3.

[81] Rau JL. Design principles of liquid nebulization devices currently in use. Respir Care 2002;47:1257–75 [discussion: 1275–78].

[82] Greenspan BJ. Ultrasonic and electrohydrodynamic methods for aerosol generation. In: Hickey AJ, editor. Inhalation aerosols: physical and biologic basis for therapy. Lung Biology in Health and Disease, vol. 94. New York: Marcel Dekker; 1996. p. 313–35.

[83] Harvey CJ, O'Doherty MJ, Page CJ, et al. Comparison of jet and ultrasonic nebulizer pulmonary aerosol deposition during mechanical ventilation. Eur Respir J 1997;10:905–9.

[84] Phillips GD, Millard FJ. The therapeutic use of ultrasonic nebulizers in acute asthma. Respir Med 1994;88:387–9.

[85] Phipps PR, Gonda I. Droplets produced by medical nebulizers. Some factors affecting their size and solute concentration. Chest 1990;97:1327–32.

[86] Steckel H, Eskandar F. Factors affecting aerosol performance during nebulization with jet and ultrasonic nebulizers. Eur J Pharm Sci 2003;19:443–55.

[87] Thomas SH, O'Doherty MJ, Page CJ, et al. Delivery of ultrasonic nebulized aerosols to a lung model during mechanical ventilation. Am Rev Respir Dis 1993;148:872–7.

[88] Dhand R. Nebulizers that use a vibrating mesh or plate with multiple apertures to generate aerosol. Respir Care 2002;47:1406–16 [discussion: 1416–18].

[89] Smaldone GC. Advances in aerosols: adult respiratory disease. J Aerosol Med 2006;19:36–46.

[90] Van Dyke RE, Nikander K. Delivery of iloprost inhalation solution with the HaloLite, Prodose, and I-neb adaptive aerosol delivery systems: an in vitro study. Respir care 2007;52(2):184–90.

[91] Waldrep JC, Berlinski A, Dhand R. Comparative analysis of methods to measure aerosols generated by a vibrating mesh nebulizer. J Aerosol Med 2007;20(3):310–9.

[92] Waldrep JC, Dhand R. Advanced nebulizer designs employing vibrating mesh/aperture plate technologies for aerosol generation. Current Drug Delivery 2008;5, in press.

[93] Dolovich MB, Ahrens RC, Hess DR, et al. Device selection and outcomes of aerosol therapy: evidence-based guidelines: American College of Chest Physicians/American College of Asthma, Allergy, and Immunology. Chest 2005;127:335–71.

[94] Craven DE, Lichtenberg DA, Goularte TA, et al. Contaminated medication nebulizers in mechanical ventilator circuits. Source of bacterial aerosols. Am J Med 1984;77:834–8.

[95] Hamill RJ, Houston ED, Georghiou PR, et al. An outbreak of Burkholderia (formerly Pseudomonas)

cepacia respiratory tract colonization and infection associated with nebulized albuterol therapy. Ann Intern Med 1995;122:762–6.

[96] Ballard J, Lugo RA, Salyer JW. A survey of albuterol administration practices in intubated patients in the neonatal intensive care unit. Respir Care 2002;47:31–8.

[97] Chang LH, Honiden S, Haithcock JA, et al. Utilization of bronchodilators in ventilated patients without obstructive airways disease. Respir Care 2007;52(2):154–8.

[98] Summer W, Elston R, Tharpe L, et al. Aerosol bronchodilator delivery methods. Relative impact on pulmonary function and cost of respiratory care. Arch Intern Med 1989;149:618–23.

[99] Bowton DL, Goldsmith WM, Haponik EF. Substitution of metered-dose inhalers for hand-held nebulizers. Success and cost savings in a large, acute-care hospital. Chest 1992;101:305–8.

[100] Ely EW, Baker AM, Evans GW, et al. The distribution of costs of care in mechanically ventilated patients with chronic obstructive pulmonary disease. Crit Care Med 2000;28:408–13.

[101] O'Riordan TG, Palmer LB, Smaldone GC. Aerosol deposition in mechanically ventilated patients. Optimizing nebulizer delivery. Am J Respir Crit Care Med 1994;149:214–9.

[102] Ahrens RC, Ries RA, Popendorf W, et al. The delivery of therapeutic aerosols through endotracheal tubes. Pediatr Pulmonol 1986;2:19–26.

[103] Newman SP. How well do in vitro particle size measurements predict drug delivery in vitro. J Aerosol Med 1998;11(1):S97–103.

[104] Lange CF, Finlay WH. Overcoming the adverse effect of humidity in aerosol delivery via pressurized metered-dose inhalers during mechanical ventilation. Am J Respir Crit Care Med 2000;161:1614–8.

[105] Wilkes AR. Heat and moisture exchangers: structure and function. Respir Care Clin N Am 1998; 4:261–79.

[106] Habib DM, Garner SS, Brandeburg S. Effect of helium-oxygen on delivery of albuterol in a pediatric, volume-cycled, ventilated lung model. Pharmacotherapy 1999;19:143–9.

[107] Goode ML, Fink JB, Dhand R, et al. Improvement in aerosol delivery with helium-oxygen mixtures during mechanical ventilation. Am J Respir Crit Care Med 2001;163:109–14.

[108] Svartengren M, Anderson M, Philipson K, et al. Human lung deposition of particles suspended in air or in helium/oxygen mixture. Exp Lung Res 1989;15(4):575–85.

[109] Anderson M, Svartengren M, Bylin G, et al. Deposition in asthmatics of particles inhaled in air or in helium-oxygen. Am J Respir Crit Care Med 1993; 147(3):524–8.

[110] Hess DR, Acosta FL, Ritz RH, et al. The effect of heliox on nebulizer function using a beta-agonist bronchodilator. Chest 1999;115:184–9.

[111] Crogan SJ, Bishop MJ. Delivery efficiency of metered dose aerosols given via endotracheal tubes. Anesthesiology 1989;70:1008–10.

[112] Dhand R. Special problems in aerosol delivery: artificial airways. Respir Care 2000;45:636–45.

[113] Fink JB, Dhand R, Duarte AG, et al. Aerosol delivery from a metered-dose inhaler during mechanical ventilation. An in vitro model. Am J Respir Crit Care Med 1996;154:382–7.

[114] Dhand R. Maximizing aerosol delivery during mechanical ventilation: go with the flow and go slow. Intensive Care Med 2003;29:1041–2.

[115] McPeck M, O'Riordan TG, Smaldone GC. Predicting aerosol delivery to intubated patients: influence of choice of mechanical ventilator on nebulizer efficiency. Respir Care 1993;38(8):887–95.

[116] Dolovich MA. Influence of inspiratory flow rate, particle size, and airway caliber on aerosolized drug delivery to the lung. Respir Care 2000;45: 597–608.

[117] Fink JB, Dhand R. Aerosol therapy in mechanically ventilated patients: recent advances and new techniques. Semin Respir Crit Care Med 2000; 21(3):183–201.

[118] Guerin C, Durand PG, Pereira C, et al. Effects of inhaled fenoterol and positive end-expiratory pressure on the respiratory mechanics of patients with chronic obstructive pulmonary disease. Can Respir J 2005;12(6):329–35.

[119] Duarte AG, Dhand R, Reid R, et al. Serum albuterol levels in mechanically ventilated patients and healthy subjects after metered-dose inhaler administration. Am J Respir Crit Care Med 1996;154: 1658–63.

[120] Marik P, Hogan J, Krikorian J. A comparison of bronchodilator therapy delivered by nebulization and metered-dose inhaler in mechanically ventilated patients. Chest 1999;115:1653–7.

[121] Newman SP, Pavia D, Morén F, et al. Deposition of pressurized aerosols in the human respiratory tract. Thorax 1981;36(1):52–5.

[122] Dolovich M, Ruffin RE, Roberts R, et al. Optimal delivery of aerosols from metered dose inhalers. Chest 1981;80(6 Suppl):911–5.

[123] Vecellio L, Guérin C, Grimbert D, et al. In vitro study and semiempirical model for aerosol delivery control during mechanical ventilation. Intensive Care Med 2005;31(6):871–6.

[124] Fink J. Aerosol drug therapy. In: Wilkins RL, Stoller JK, Scanlan CL, editors. Egan's fundamentals of respiratory care. 8th edition. St. Louis (MO): Mosby; 2003. p. 761–800.

[125] Boucher BA, Kuhl DA, Coffey BC, et al. Drug use in a trauma intensive-care unit. Am J Hosp Pharm 1990;151:1827–33.

[126] Wollam PJ, Kasper CL, Bishop MJ, et al. Prediction and assessment of bronchodilator response in mechanically ventilated patients. Respir Care 1994;39:730–5.

[127] Gay PC, Rodarte JR, Tayyab M, et al. Evaluation of bronchodilator responsiveness in mechanically ventilated patients. Am Rev Respir Dis 1987;136: 880–5.

[128] Wright PE, Carmichael LC, Bernard GR. Effect of bronchodilators on lung mechanics in the acute respiratory distress syndrome (ARDS). Chest 1994;106:1517–23.

[129] Morina P, Herrera M, Venegas J, et al. Effects of nebulized salbutamol on respiratory mechanics in adult respiratory distress syndrome. Intensive Care Med 1997;23:58–64.

[130] Mancebo J, Amaro P, Lorino H, et al. Effects of albuterol inhalation on the work of breathing during weaning from mechanical ventilation. Am Rev Respir Dis 1991;144(1):95–100.

[131] Bennett WD. Effect of beta-adrenergic agonists on mucociliary clearance. J Allergy Clin Immunol 2002;110:S291–7.

[132] McAuley DF, Frank JA, Fang X, et al. Clinically relevant concentrations of beta2-adrenergic agonists stimulate maximal cyclic adenosine monophosphate-dependent airspace fluid clearance and decrease pulmonary edema in experimental acid-induced lung injury. Crit Care Med 2004;32(7): 1470–6.

[133] Fernandez A, Munoz J, de la Calle B, et al. Comparison of one versus two bronchodilators in ventilated COPD patients. Intensive Care Med 1994;20: 199–202.

[134] Abramson MJ, Walters J, Walters EH. Adverse effects of beta-agonists: are they clinically relevant? Am J Respir Med 2003;2(4):287–97.

[135] Kleerup EC, Tashkin DP, Cline AC, et al. Cumulative dose-response study of non-CFC propellant HFA-134a salbutamol sulfate metered-dose inhaler in patients with asthma. Chest 1996;109:702–7.

[136] Ramsdell JW, Colice GL, Ekholm BP, et al. Cumulative dose response study comparing HFA-134a albuterol sulfate and conventional CFC albuterol in patients with asthma. Ann Allergy Asthma Immunol 1998;81:593–9.

[137] Dhand R. Bronchodilator therapy in mechanically ventilated patients: patient selection and clinical outcomes. Respir Care 2007;52(2):152–3.

[138] Carlucci A, Richard JC, Wysocki M, et al. Noninvasive versus conventional mechanical ventilation: an epidemiologic survey. Am J Respir Crit Care Med 2001;163:874–80.

[139] Brochard L, Mancebo J, Wysocki M, et al. Noninvasive ventilation for acute exacerbations of chronic obstructive pulmonary disease. N Engl J Med 1995;333(13):817–22.

[140] Bott J, Carroll MP, Conway JH, et al. Randomised controlled trial of nasal ventilation in acute ventilatory failure due to chronic obstructive airways disease. Lancet 1993;341(8860):1555–7.

[141] Kramer N, Meyer TJ, Meharg J, et al. Randomized, prospective trial of noninvasive positive pressure ventilation in acute respiratory failure. Am J Respir Crit Care Med 1995;151(6):1799–806.

[142] Ram FS, Picot J, Lightowler J, et al. Non-invasive positive pressure ventilation for treatment of respiratory failure due to exacerbations of chronic obstructive pulmonary disease. Cochrane Database Syst Rev 2004;(3):CD004104.

[143] Ferrer M, Valencia M, Nicolas JM, et al. Early noninvasive ventilation averts extubation failure in patients at risk: a randomized trial. Am J Respir Crit Care Med 2006;173(2):164–70.

[144] Shenfield GM, Evans ME, Walker SR, et al. The fate of nebulized salbutamol (albuterol) administered by intermittent positive pressure respiration to asthmatic patients. Am Rev Respir Dis 1973; 108(3):501–5.

[145] Parkes SN, Bersten AD. Aerosol kinetics and bronchodilator efficacy during continuous positive airway pressure delivered by face mask. Thorax 1997;52(2):171–5.

[146] Dolovich MB, Killian D, Wolff RK, et al. Pulmonary aerosol deposition in chronic bronchitis: intermittent positive pressure breathing versus quiet breathing. Am Rev Respir Dis 1977;115(3):397–402.

[147] Hess DR. The mask for noninvasive ventilation: principles of design and effects on aerosol delivery. J Aerosol Med 2007;20(Suppl 1):S85–99.

[148] Chatmongkolchart S, Schettino GP, Dillman C, et al. In vitro evaluation of aerosol bronchodilator delivery during noninvasive positive pressure ventilation: effect of ventilator settings and nebulizer position. Crit Care Med 2002;30(11):2515–9.

[149] Fauroux B, Itti E, Pigeot J, et al. Optimization of aerosol deposition by pressure support in children with cystic fibrosis: an experimental and clinical study. Am J Respir Crit Care Med 2000;162(6): 2265–71.

[150] Branconnier MP, Hess DR. Albuterol delivery during noninvasive ventilation. Respir Care 2005; 50(12):1649–53.

[151] Nava S, Karakurt S, Rampulla C, et al. Salbutamol delivery during non-invasive mechanical ventilation in patients with chronic obstructive pulmonary disease: a randomized, controlled study. Intensive Care Med 2001;27(10):1627–35.

[152] Pollack CV Jr, Fleisch KB, Dowsey K. Treatment of acute bronchospasm with beta-adrenergic agonist aerosols delivered by a nasal bilevel positive airway pressure circuit. Ann Emerg Med 1995; 26(5):552–7.

[153] Jolliet P, Tassaux D, Roeseler J, et al. Helium-oxygen versus air-oxygen noninvasive pressure support in decompensated chronic obstructive disease: a prospective, multicenter study. Crit Care Med 2003;31(3):878–84.

ELSEVIER
SAUNDERS

Clin Chest Med 29 (2008) 297–312

CLINICS
IN CHEST
MEDICINE

Do Newer Monitors of Exhaled Gases, Mechanics, and Esophageal Pressure Add Value?

Robert L. Owens, MD[a,b], William S. Stigler, MD[b,c],
Dean R. Hess, PhD, RRT[b,d],*

[a]Department of Medicine, Pulmonary and Critical Care Unit, Cox 2, Massachusetts General Hospital,
55 Fruit Street, Boston, MA 02114, USA
[b]Harvard Medical School, Boston, MA, USA
[c]Massachusetts General Hospital, 15 Parkman Street, Wang Ambulatory Care Center 645, Boston, MA 02114, USA
[d]Respiratory Care, Ellison 401, Massachusetts General Hospital, 55 Fruit Street, Boston, MA 02114, USA

When introduced into widespread use in the 1950s, mechanical ventilation reduced mortality attributable to respiratory failure. However, it was later recognized that in addition to this life-saving potential, mechanical ventilation could be injurious to the lung and further cause widespread organ failure [1]. Ventilator-induced lung injury (VILI) is proposed to occur through at least two mechanisms: end-inspiratory alveolar over-distension (volutrauma) and end-expiratory alveolar derecruitment (atelectrauma), caused by repeated opening and closing during tidal ventilation [2]. The recognition of VILI and these mechanisms has driven clinicians to seek a balance between over-distension and derecruitment. While lung protective strategies as advocated by the Acute Respiratory Distress Syndrome Network (ARDS-Net) and others have demonstrated benefit in mortality, there is indirect evidence that these strategies may not benefit all patients. Examples include radiographic findings of alveolar over-distension using the ARDSNet ventilatory strategy of 6-mL/kg predicted body weight, and failure to demonstrate a mortality benefit for a higher positive end-expiratory pressure (PEEP) strategy in the ALVEOLI (Assessment of Low Tidal Volume and Elevated End Expiratory Volume to Obviate Lung Injury) trial [3,4]. These findings

suggest potential benefit for individualized, dynamic assessment of lung mechanics and real-time ventilator management based on underlying pathophysiology. This article addresses whether measures of lung inflammation and mechanics are a beneficial component of a lung protective ventilatory strategy.

Exhaled breath condensate

Exhaled breath condensate (EBC) offers a non-invasive method of monitoring disease through the measurement of various components present within exhaled breath. The most investigated components of EBC are pH and the quantitative measurement of several biomarkers, including exhaled nitrogen oxide compounds, leukotrienes, isoprostanes, hydrogen peroxide, and cytokines. These components have been evaluated in a variety of pulmonary processes including chronic obstructive pulmonary disease (COPD), asthma, acute lung injury (ALI), and pneumonia.

Despite these studies, the anatomic origin of EBC is unclear. If from multiple sources, the relative contributions of the components of the respiratory tract have not been elucidated. Furthermore, different components of EBC will arise from different parts of the respiratory system: aerosolized particles likely arise from alveoli or areas of turbulent flow, while volatile compounds could arise from the entire airway [5]. Because EBC is a sample of the entire respiratory system, it does not only reflect lower airways. Thus,

* Corresponding author. Respiratory Care, Ellison 401, Massachusetts General Hospital, 55 Fruit Street, Boston, MA 02114.

E-mail address: dhess@partners.org (D.R. Hess).

concentrations of EBC markers do not correlate with those found in bronchoalveolar lavage (BAL) [6,7]. Study designs also include testing samples for amylase to exclude oropharyngeal contamination (although during mechanical ventilation, oropharyngeal contamination should be minimal if the patient is intubated). Nevertheless, proponents argue that EBC is a potentially useful marker of inflammation, lung injury, and alveolar over-distension that is easily obtainable.

Measurement and technical difficulties

The basic method of collection involves the patient breathing normal tidal volumes, with the exhaled breath traveling through a condensing system. The time for collection varies, but on average requires 10 to 15 minutes to obtain a sufficient sample size. There are two commercially available devices, the RTube (Respiratory Research, Inc., Charlottesville, Virginia) and ECoScreen (VIASYS Health care, Yorba Linda, California) (Fig. 1). The RTube is a disposable collection system consisting of a mouthpiece, saliva trap, collection tube, and cooling sleeve. The sleeve is cooled by a freezer to −20°C and is

then placed around the collection tube. The ECoScreen uses a constant temperature condenser (−15°C). Comparison between these two devices shows differences in collection volumes and mediator recovery [8]. EBC was collected from 30 healthy adults using both devices consecutively, in random sequence. Mean volume and concentrations of some biomarkers collected using the ECoScreen were significantly higher when compared with the RTube; however, there was no difference between median pH. The authors hypothesize that the difference in collection volume is because of temperature changes of the condensing systems during collection. The RTube, because it is cooled before collection, equilibrates with the environment and warms during measurement; the ECoScreen is maintained at a constant temperature during collection. However, additional studies suggest that pH does vary significantly between devices, with the RTube collection system providing a more acidic EBC [9].

These studies highlight the difficulty comparing studies of EBC. There is not yet a single standard method for collection. Prior to commercially produced devices, researchers created condensing units for the collection of EBC. Given the

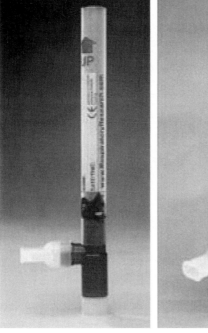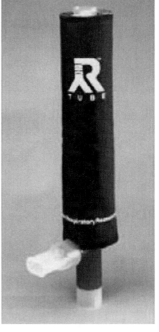

Fig. 1. The R-Tube, a commercially available device for exhaled breath condensate. The handheld device includes a side mouthpiece, a saliva trap, and a collecting tube. The collecting tube is surrounded by a cold metal sleeve during sample collection. (*Courtesy of* Respiratory Research, Inc., Charlottesville, VA; with permission.)

apparent variability between the devices described above in regards to temperature of condensing sleeve, collection volume, biomarkers, and pH, it stands to reason that a similar variability would exist between more individualized devices. These differences do not negate significant findings but make it more difficult to create normative data in regards to the components of EBC. One mitigating factor is that intermeasurement variability between adult subjects using the RTube collection system appears minimal. A study of inter- and intra-day variability from 21 volunteers showed a high level of reproducibility. The variables measured were pH, protein content, and volume. The only significant difference noted was that an initial collection netted a sample of lower volume and protein content; this is likely explained by inexperienced subjects, as it was not seen in those subjects who had experience with EBC collection [10]. Also, while the volume of collection increases with minute ventilation, concentrations of markers or pH are not altered [11]. Finally, EBC has been studied in subjects with acute asthma exacerbation, and can be performed easily and safely [12].

As with nonventilated patients, no standard exists for the collection of EBC in mechanically ventilated patients. When performed, EBC collection is obtained through the expiratory limb of the ventilator tubing attached to one of the commercial collecting units. One older study simply placed the tubing though an ice bath [13]. There are few studies of the relationship of disease and concentration of red blood cell markers in the mechanically ventilated patient (see below). Hindering clinical use of EBC is the lack of normative data. There are currently no normal reference values, except for recent attempts to establish reference ranges for EBC pH in healthy adults [14,15].

Specific biomarkers in mechanical ventilation

Nitric oxide

Nitric oxide (NO) is a free radical that reacts rapidly with reactive oxygen species and is itself difficult to measure. However, some metabolites are more stable, such as NO_2^- (nitrite) and NO_3^- (nitrate). These nonvolatile compounds have been investigated in several clinical settings, such as in patients with obstructive lung disease and cigarette smokers. As compared with healthy nonsmokers, NO_3^- levels are higher in asymptomatic smokers, asthmatics, and patients with

community acquired pneumonia [16]. NO_2^- is more closely linked to COPD and hyperinflation. Gessner and colleagues [17] found that NO_2^- concentration in EBC correlates with residual volume (RV), total lung capacity (TLC), intrathoracic gas volume, and the RV/TLC ratio. In the same analysis, NO_2^- levels were not related to inflammatory cytokines in EBC. The inestigators hypothesize that NO_2^- is not a marker of inflammation but instead is related to mechanical stretch and hyperinflation. Further evidence suggesting that NO_2^- is a marker of alveolar distension comes from mechanically ventilated patients. In patients with and without ALI, NO_2^- level correlated with tidal volume. Again, no correlation was found with other inflammatory markers, suggesting that NO_2^- may be a specific marker of alveolar overdistension [18].

pH

Low EBC pH was first noted in asthma exacerbations and more recently has been implicated in other pulmonary disorders, including COPD, bronchiectasis, and ARDS [19–21]. Acidic pH has generally been thought to be a marker of airways inflammation; however, it may also act to worsen bronchoconstriction, impair ciliary motility, increase mucus viscosity, and induce epithelial damage [22–25]. As a marker of inflammation in acute lung injury, EBC pH was studied by Gessner and colleagues [21]. Using a continuous pH probe, they found that EBC pH had an inverse relationship to Lung Index Severity Score and EBC proinflammatory cytokines, such as interleukin (IL)-6 and IL-8. In patients monitored continuously, changes in pH have also been studied. Decreases in pH preceded a subsequent clinical deterioration in a diverse group of pediatric patients with respiratory failure [26]. Conversely, a rise in pH has been observed in response to treatment in asthmatic patients [27].

Isoprostanes

Isoprostanes are a novel class of compounds formed by in vivo lipid peroxidation of membrane arachindonic acid. It appears these serve as markers of airway inflammation, similar to EBC pH. In the setting of oxidant stress, 8-iso-prostaglandin F2a is elevated, and in 22 subjects with ARDS was significantly elevated in EBC as compared with controls [13]. Their use as a marker of airway inflammation is supported by isoprostane elevation in the EBC of COPD patients experiencing exacerbation [28]. Notably, the levels of

8-isoprostane decreased significantly within 2 weeks of initiating therapy with antibiotics.

Hydrogen peroxide

Hydrogen peroxide (H_2O_2) is a nonvolatile reactive oxygen species that plays a central role in forming cytotoxic hydroxyl radicals shown to be a marker of airway inflammation. An example is the elevation of H_2O_2 in pneumonia related to the influx of phagocytic cells in the lower airways [29]. H_2O_2 concentration also correlates with induced sputum eosinophil count [30]. There is limited data for measurements of H_2O_2 in the critically ill, though H_2O_2 concentrations do correlate with severity of ARDS [31,32].

Conclusion

The clinical utility of monitoring of exhaled breath is unknown at this time. Even allowing that EBC contents might be specific markers of over-distension, inflammation, or infection, no trial to date has incorporated EBC into a ventilatory strategy. In general, the use of EBC in the clinical setting will require: better understanding of the anatomic region of the respiratory tract from which a particular marker arises; its clinical significance in specific diseases; reasonable turn-around time on results and; proof that using these results improves a clinically significant outcome. One would hope, for example, to use EBC nitrates as a marker for alveolar over-distension in real time. However, at this time, none of the currently studied markers meet these criteria.

Mechanics

Unlike EBC, lung mechanics have been studied for decades in a variety of settings in an attempt to balance alveolar derecruitment and over-distension. Furthermore, several methods of incorporating lung mechanics into a ventilatory strategy have been used in clinical trials.

Pressure-volume curves

One proposed mechanism for monitoring lung mechanics is the quasistatic pressure-volume curve (P-V curve). In healthy adult subjects, the P-V curve has a sigmoidal shape and reflects the balance of forces between the lung and chest wall. With inflation beginning at residual volume, the curve initially exhibits a segment with low compliance, followed by a linear region with high compliance, and finally a low compliance segment. The shape of the P-V curve represents the

low compliance of the chest wall at low lung volumes and the low compliance of the lungs at high lung volumes in normal subjects.

In patients with ALI, the P-V curve has a sigmoidal shape beginning with inflation from functional residual capacity (Figs. 2 and 3). In this case, the three regions of the curve are thought to represent three distinct phases of alveolar state: derecruited, collapsed alveoli at low lung volumes; recruitment and "balloon-like" filling at moderate lung volumes; and over-distension at high lung volumes. The intersections of these regions have been called the lower inflection point (LIP) and the upper inflection point (UIP). Because the LIP was thought to represent alveolar recruitment, it was advocated as an appropriate pressure to set PEEP. The UIP was thought to represent the point of over-distension and was thus used to determine a safe upper limit of alveolar distending pressure.

In ventilated patients with ALI, P-V curves have been used diagnostically and to guide ventilator management. Bone [33] used P-V curves to diagnose causes of respiratory failure and to assess response to therapy. A hallmark of ALI is reduced lung compliance, reflected as a shift in the P-V curve to the right. Also in ALI, Matamis

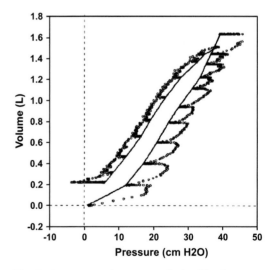

Fig. 2. A pressure-volume curve obtained by the super-syringe method. Open circles represent points obtained continuously during the maneuver. The solid line is interpolated data between quasi-static equilibration points. Note the changes in pressure with each volume change, representing airway resistance and then stress relaxation. (*From* Harris RS. Pressure-volume curves of the respiratory system. Respir Care 2005;50(1):78–98; discussion 98–9; with permission.)

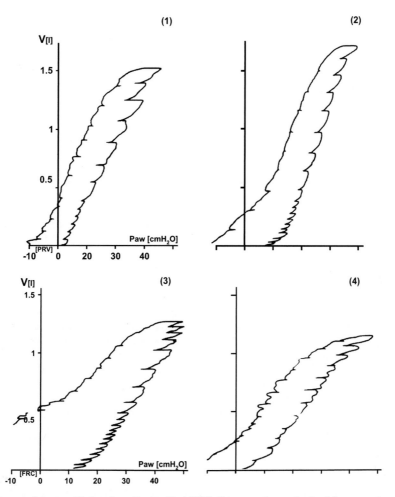

Fig. 3. The P-V curve changes with time in patients with ARDS. Curve no. 1 was obtained from a patient after recovery from ARDS, and appears normal. Curve no. 2 early in ARDS, with only alveolar opacities seen on chest X-ray, demonstrates normal compliance, but with the appearance of a lower inflection point. As ARDS progresses to include interstitial opacities on chest X-ray (curve no. 3), and then to a later fibroproliferative stage (curve no. 4), the P-V curve shifts to the right, consistent with reduced compliance. (*From* Matamis D, Lemaire F, Harf A, et al. Total respiratory pressure-volume curves in the adult respiratory distress syndrome. Chest 1984;86(1):58–66; with permission.)

and colleagues [34] showed a correlation between shift in the P-V curve and the radiographic severity of ARDS. Suter and Dall'ava-Santucci focused on the lower inflection point, and suggested that it is best to set PEEP at or just above this point [35,36]. Using this hypothesis, Amato and colleagues [37] incorporated P-V curves into a lung protective ventilatory strategy. One key feature of this strategy was low tidal volume ventilation; however, a small tidal volume may increase the risk for derecruitment unless an appropriate level of PEEP is applied. Thus, the lower inflection point was assessed and PEEP was set just above this pressure ("Pflex" plus 2 cm H_2O). Patients

treated with this lung protective ventilatory strategy, compared with a traditional ventilation strategy, had a lower mortality at 28 days, more rapid weaning from mechanical ventilation, and less barotrauma. Ranieri and colleagues [38] used P-V curves in a lung protective ventilation strategy and reported lower cytokine concentrations in the BAL and plasma when compared with patients undergoing conventional ventilation. A recent similar trial using lower tidal volumes with PEEP set above the lower inflection point also demonstrated a clinical benefit [39]. However, despite the interest that these studies have generated for the use of the P-V curve to determine mechanical ventilator settings, a variety of theoretic and practical concerns have limited their acceptance and use.

What does the P-V curve tell us about the alveoli?

The clinical trials discussed above assume that the P-V curve, a measurement performed at the airway opening, reflects the performance of individual alveoli. In reality, the P-V curve is an aggregate of all alveoli. New models of the P-V curve, as well as indirect and direct visualization of alveoli, have increased our understanding of alveolar function in ALI and how it relates to the P-V curve. Hickling [40] modeled the lungs with ARDS and predicted alveolar recruitment along the entire length of the P-V curve. As a result, a PEEP setting much higher than the LIP is needed for full alveolar recruitment. A clinical study by Jonson and colleagues [41] confirmed additional recruitment at pressures above the LIP and along the entire inflation P-V curve. Similar findings have been observed from CT images and microscopy [42,43]. These studies call into question the concept that alveolar recruitment occurs at or near the lower inflection point.

What does the P-V curve tell us about the chest wall?

Another assumption implicit in the clinical use of the P-V curve is that it reflects the mechanical characteristics of the lungs. However, the P-V curve obtained at the airway opening includes contributions from the lungs and the chest wall. The chest wall includes the thoracic cage and diaphragm, which is affected by intra-abdominal pressure. It has been shown that chest wall mechanics can influence the P-V curve of the total respiratory system [44,45]. Ranieri and colleagues [45] reported that in patients with ARDS related to major abdominal surgery (surgical ARDS), the inspiratory P-V curve of the respiratory system and lungs showed an upward convexity, indicating that compliance decreased with inflation. Patients with ARDS not consequent to major surgery (medical ARDS) had an upward concavity on the inspiratory P-V curves of the respiratory system and lungs, indicating an increase in compliance and alveolar recruitment with lung inflation. This suggests that the flattening of the P-V curve of the respiratory system observed in some patients with ARDS may be because of a decrease in chest wall compliance related to abdominal distension. If chest wall effects are not considered, unnecessary restriction of tidal volume might

occur in patients with surgical ARDS, and overestimation of the PEEP requirement might occur in patients with medical ARDS (Fig. 4).

Mergoni and colleagues [44] also studied the effects of chest-wall mechanics on the respiratory system P-V curve in patients with acute respiratory failure. They found that the improvement in PaO_2 with PEEP is significant only in patients in whom the lower inflection point is on the lung P-V curve and not on the chest wall P-V curve. As a result, these investigators have advocated measurement of lung mechanics alone (rather than those of the total respiratory system) to set PEEP and other ventilator settings. Whether this makes clinical sense, as the lung is not ventilated in isolation, remains unknown. The lung and chest wall components are frequently separated with esophageal balloon manometry, which may provide further information (see below).

Inflation versus deflation curves

The inflation limb of the P-V curve has been most commonly used to determine ventilator settings in investigations of patients with ARDS. However, several studies call into question the use of Pflex on the inflation limb to set PEEP. PEEP is used to prevent alveolar collapse on deflation. Thus, it would seem that the deflation limb would be best for identifying the end-expiratory pressure to prevent collapse [46–49]. In patients with ARDS, Holzapfel and colleagues [47] compared the reduction in shunt fraction with the inflation and deflation P-V curves as PEEP was progressively increased. The maximum reduction in shunt correlated best with the true inflection point (the point where concavity changes direction) of the deflation P-V curve. In anesthetized patients, nitrogen washout studies have shown that the deflation limb of the P-V curve can be used to estimate the pressure required to raise functional residual capacity (FRC) above closing volume [50]. Using mathematical models, alveolar collapse occurs at a pressure greater than the true inflection point [51].

Because lung volume is greater for a given level of PEEP on the deflation limb—compared with the inflation limb—of the P-V curve, recent attention has been given to full alveolar inflation using a recruitment maneuver, followed by a decremental PEEP trial. It is hoped that this will result in ventilation on the deflation limb, but outcome studies are lacking to support this approach. Albaiceta and colleagues [52] studied the effects of two levels of PEEP: 2 cm H_2O above

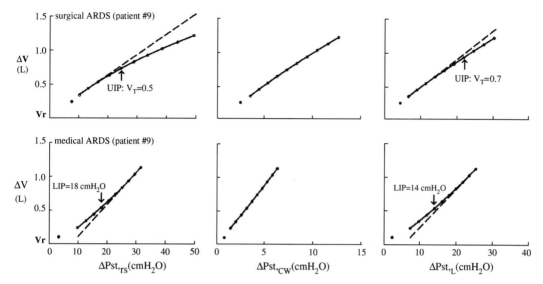

Fig. 4. The chest wall in ARDS. Alterations in chest wall compliance may contribute substantially to the mechanics of the total respiratory system. Shown here are two representative pressure volume curves of the total respiratory system, the chest wall, and the lung alone from patients with surgical and medical ARDS. The surgical patient has a greater decrease in chest wall compliance. Whether LIP or UIP should be measured from the total respiratory system or the lung alone is not known. (*From* Ranieri VM, Brienza N, Santostasi S, et al. Impairment of lung and chest wall mechanics in patients with acute respiratory distress syndrome: role of abdominal distension. Am J Respir Crit Care Med 1997;156(4 Pt 1):1082–91; with permission.)

the lower inflection point of the inflation limb and equal to the point of maximum curvature on the deflation limb of the P-V curve. PEEP, according to the point of maximum curvature on the deflation limb, was related to an improvement in oxygenation, decrease in nonaerated lung volumes, and greater alveolar stability. However, there was also an increase in $PaCO_2$, airway pressures, and hyperaerated lung volume.

Measurement and technical difficulties

There are a number of technical challenges in the acquisition and interpretation of P-V curves that limit their clinical use. There is no single technique used to obtain the curve and this may affect clinical interpretation. With the super-syringe method, after the lung reaches a relaxation volume, serial aliquots of oxygen (100 mL–200 mL each) are injected into the lungs and airway pressure is measured after 2 to 3 seconds of equilibration at each volume. Volume is added until some arbitrary airway pressure is reached (for example, 40 cm H_2O). While relatively easy to perform, this method requires extra equipment, opening of the ventilator circuit, and the patient must be heavily sedated or paralyzed. The relatively long time required to perform the entire procedure means that the curves

must be adjusted for gas exchange that takes place during the measurement [53]. Decailliot and colleagues [54] reported that P-V curves can be obtained without paralysis in some patients. However, this was not feasible in a significant minority of patients and they concluded that, "the level of intra-individual variability in measurements indicates that P-V curve without paralysis should be used with caution at the bedside for clinical management." Lee and colleagues [55] obtained serial P-V curves in subjects with ARDS using the syringe method and found it safe for most patients, although some subjects did have changes in hemodynamics or oxygenation, and the study was discontinued in 2 out of 11 subjects. Similar results were reported by Roch and colleagues [56].

Concerns related to the clinical use of the super-syringe method generated interest in "quasi-static" P-V curves. For example, the constant-flow method uses a low gas flow (less than 10 L per minute) to inflate the lungs as pressure at the proximal airway is measured. The multiple-occlusion technique measures end-inspiratory occlusion pressures with different inflation volumes; the result is that the data points to construct a P-V curve. Both methods avoid ventilator disconnection and do not require additional equipment.

However, both require sedation or paralysis as they involve slow flow rates (to minimize airway resistance effects) and breath holds, respectively [57]. To avoid these problems, some investigators have advocated the use of the "dynostatic pressure," a method of measuring alveolar pressure across a range of volumes to construct an approximation of the static P-V curve during therapeutic mechanical ventilation [58–62]. Assuming inspiratory and expiratory resistances are equal (which is often not a correct assumption), alveolar pressure is calculated from intratracheal pressure and the dynostatic P-V curve is constructed. Note that this curve is a composite of the inflation and deflation curves. These methods, while advantageous in some ways, have not been as rigorously studied, compared with P-V curves generated from the super-syringe method.

Others have advocated the use of "dynamic" P-V curves, obtained by measuring static compliance across a range of PEEP settings. This can be performed automatically without additional sedation or significant ventilator setting changes. However, there is not good agreement between static and dynamic P-V curves [63,64]. Stahl and colleagues [64] argue that the difference arises because dynamic measurements only reflect the intra-tidal mechanics and are not influenced by recruitment across the entire P-V curve. They suggest that dynamic P-V curves are more sensitive for assessing intra-tidal over-distension or recruitment/derecruitment, and thus should be used to establish safe ventilation parameters. However, dynamic P-V curves have not been used in clinical outcome trials or correlated with alveolar function with imaging or microscopy. Whether the dynamic P-V curve provides additional information

beyond that obtained from a pressure-time curve (see below), which may be easier to measure, is also not known.

Assuming the P-V curve is constructed of either the lungs alone or the total respiratory system, or whether using a static or dynamic method, there is still considerable variation in interpretation. Harris and colleagues [65] showed that there was significant inter- and intra-observer variability in determining Pflex. Given the range of pressures for LIP and UIP identified by clinicians from visual inspection of the curves, this likely represented clinically important differences if the data were used to set PEEP. The application of a rigorous mathematic model proposed by Venegas may help reduce some of the errors in both terminology and observer variability [66].

How do ventilators generate P-V curves?

Most current generation adult mechanical ventilators have the capability to display P-V loops. However, one must avoid the temptation to simply display these loops, identify inflection points, and then set the ventilator accordingly. P-V loops generated during ventilation do not fulfill the condition of zero flow; gas flow generates an additional pressure because of airway resistance. Moreover, the flow during inhalation is often not constant (eg, pressure controlled ventilation, descending ramp volume-controlled ventilation), and the flow during passive exhalation is exponential. In addition, active breathing efforts by the patient invalidate the P-V curve. During pressure-controlled ventilation, for example, the P-V is typically box-shaped (Fig. 5) and characteristics of this loop more closely reflect how the ventilator is set than the underlying pathophysiology of the lungs.

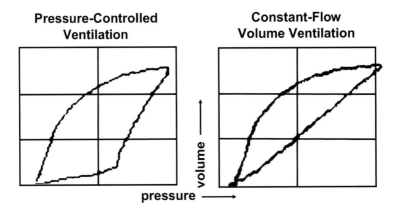

Fig. 5. Pressure-volume loops as typically displayed on a ventilator monitor. These curves derive their shape both from the respiratory system mechanics, and the ventilator settings.

Manufacturers of several newer ventilators have attempted to overcome these shortcomings. Most of these approaches use a low constant flow technique to allow measurement of the P-V curve with little effect of airways resistance. The curve is measured without disconnecting the patient. Typically, the user can set parameters such as flow, starting pressure, maximum pressure, and maximum volume. On some ventilators, both inflation and deflation curves can be measured (eg, Draeger, Hamilton), whereas others (eg, Viasys) only measure the inflation curve. The ventilator displays the inflection points, although the methodology used is unclear and likely proprietary, but a cursor can be used to identify the inflection points if desired. Because a constant slow flow is used that prolongs inflation, patient sedation is required. The Engstrom ventilator (GE Health care) uses a technique called SpiroDynamics, which is based on the dynostatic model detailed above. There has been little clinical validation of these approaches, such a comparison to the super-syringe technique. There also has been no head-to-head comparison to determine whether the inflection points identified by these ventilators are equivalent. Finally, whether these approaches lead to better patient outcomes is yet to be determined.

Conclusion

The P-V curve has been studied for 30 years and it has been used in clinical practice. However, our understanding of what the curve means, and how it might be used to guide ventilator management, remains incomplete. Recent studies call into question the traditional model of the P-V curve in patients with ALI/ARDS. Technical difficulties and interpretation of data also limit its clinical use.

Pressure-time curves and stress index

Another measure of respiratory system mechanics is analysis of the pressure-time (P-t) curve. This is another method to estimate lung compliance across the range of tidal breathing. Unlike P-V curves, the P-t curve can be easily measured without additional equipment or ventilator circuit disconnects, and may have less variability in interpretation. Although this curve is commonly displayed on modern ventilators, a detailed analysis of it is usually not appreciated at the bedside. The major assumption in this model is that, under constant flow conditions, resistance is constant across lung volumes. With this assumption, the rate of change in pressure with constant flow reflects compliance. It is hypothesized that concave up P-t curves represent decreasing compliance with inflation caused by tidal hyperinflation of ventilated regions. Conversely, concave down P-t curves represent increasing compliance with inflation, suggesting recruitment with tidal inflation (Fig. 6). The P-t curve can be fitted to a mathematic equation that yields a dimensionless coefficient: the stress index. A stress index value of 1 reflects constant compliance with inflation,

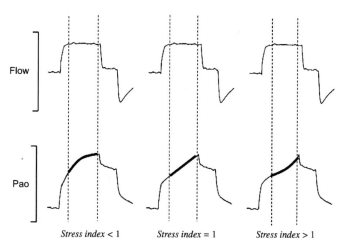

Stress index < 1   *Stress index = 1*   *Stress index > 1*

Fig. 6. The pressure-time curve and the stress index. The top figure shows essentially indistinguishable flow characteristics during assisted breathing in three different patients. The bottom figure shows the differences possible in the corresponding pressure versus time curves, with examples of stress indices below, equal to, and above 1. (*From* Grasso S, Stripoli T, De Michele M, et al. ARDSnet ventilatory protocol and alveolar hyperinflation: role of positive end-expiratory pressure. Am J Respir Crit Care Med 2007;176(8):761–7; with permission.)

less than 1 represents increasing compliance with inflation (recruitment), and greater than 1 represents decreasing compliance (hyperinflation).

Ranieri and colleagues [67] used an ex-vivo rat model of ARDS ventilated below, at, and above a stress index of 1 to assess for differences in histologic measures of lung injury and inflammatory markers. The lungs ventilated at a stress index of 1 showed the least direct evidence of lung injury and had less inflammatory cytokine production. This was validated by Grasso and colleagues [68], who compared similar ventilation strategies with CT imaging. When the stress index was less than 1, tidal ventilation showed recruitment; when it was greater than 1 there was tidal hyperinflation. Again, the hope is that a stress index value of 1 can be used to define a state of pulmonary mechanics that avoids atelectrauma and volutrauma.

Very preliminary work with the stress index has been performed in human beings by Grasso and colleagues [69]. They ventilated patients with ARDS according to the ARDSNet protocol (and lower PEEP protocol) or the ARDSNet protocol with PEEP determined by the stress index. The ARDSNet low tidal volume/PEEP protocol produced tidal hyperinflation: that is, a stress index greater than 1. Cytokine levels potentially indicating biotrauma were lower in the group managed with a PEEP set according to the stress index. This study provides information on the feasibility and ease of these measurements. The investigators report that most measurements could be made at moderate sedation levels, with only a minority of patients requiring a transient increase to a Ramsay score of 5. No paralysis was necessary; however, constant-flow volume ventilation (rather than pressure-controlled ventilation) and absence of active breathing (as opposed to pressure support ventilation) are necessary for valid measurements.

Conclusion

The stress index is a dynamic measurement of tidal changes in compliance. It has the advantage of being a bedside maneuver that requires minimal changes in ventilation (provided the patient is receiving constant flow volume ventilation), minimal changes in sedation, and appears relatively simple to reproduce and interpret. Animal studies and very early human studies demonstrate its potential benefit. That said, no automated systems to calculate the stress index are available commercially.

Esophageal manometry

The contributions of the lungs and the chest wall to respiratory mechanics can be separated with the use of esophageal balloon manometry. With this technique, a balloon-tipped catheter attached to a pressure transducer is introduced into the lower esophagus, adjacent to the pleura, and used to measure esophageal pressure as an indirect measurement of pleural pressure. Proponents argue that this allows the most accurate measurement of the transpulmonary pressure (the difference between the pressure applied at the airway and the pleural pressure); this is the distending force on the alveoli. To prevent alveolar collapse on exhalation, the transpulmonary pressure should be positive. Not only will esophageal manometry allow measurement of chest wall mechanics, but it may also be useful in determination of auto-PEEP and work of breathing.

Determination of chest wall compliance

There has been recent interest in the role of the chest wall during mechanical ventilation in critically ill patients. Chest wall compliance can be affected by a variety of conditions, including skeletal deformity, burns with escar, morbid obesity, chest wall edema, ascites, pregnancy, and abdominal compartment syndrome. In mechanically ventilated patients with acute lung injury, intra-abdominal pressure is an important determinant of chest wall compliance. Calculation of chest wall compliance requires measurements of tidal volume (V_T) and pleural pressure. Pleural pressure changes are estimated from esophageal pressure. Chest wall compliance is calculated from V_T and the corresponding change in esophageal pressure (ΔP_{eso}) (Fig. 7):

$$\text{Chest wall compliance} = V_T/\Delta P_{eso}$$

Note that estimates of pleural pressure to calculate chest wall compliance require that the patient is relaxed and breathing in synchrony with the ventilator.

In mechanical ventilated patients, Talmor and colleagues [70] used esophageal manometry and reported relatively high pleural pressures (average of 17.5 cm H_2O) in patients with acute respiratory failure. Additionally, transpulmonary pressures were sometimes negative during exhalation. From these observations, the investigators concluded that chest wall mechanics substantially influence ventilator mechanics in acute lung injury,

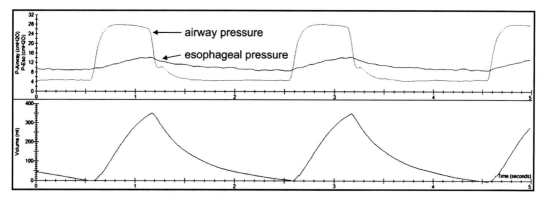

Fig. 7. Measurement of chest wall compliance with use of esophageal manometry. The top half of the figure shows esophageal pressure versus time overlayed with airway pressure, and the bottom half of the figure shows volume versus time. With inflation, both airway pressure and also esophageal pressure rise. In this example, tidal volume is 350 mL, the change in esophageal pressure is 5 cm H_2O. Thus, the chest wall compliance is 70 mL/cm H_2O.

but in an unpredictable way. They recommend further clinical study to determine if esophageal manometry can be used to individualize ventilator settings.

Detection of auto-PEEP

Auto-PEEP is most commonly quantified using an end-expiratory pause method. By imposing a period of zero flow at end-exhalation, pressure at the proximal airway approximates end-expiratory alveolar pressure. If the pressure measured during this maneuver is greater than the PEEP setting, auto-PEEP is present. A limitation of this method is that it requires passive ventilation: in other words, the patient cannot be actively breathing.

If the patient is actively breathing, esophageal pressure can be used to estimate the amount of auto-PEEP. Because auto-PEEP represents a threshold load at the beginning of inhalation, the decrease in pleural pressure (as reflected by a decrease in esophageal pressure) required to produce a positive flow at the proximal airway is the amount of auto-PEEP present (Fig. 8) [71]. In patients with spontaneous respiratory activity, recruitment of the expiratory muscles frequently generates auto-PEEP. This expiratory muscle recruitment results in a measurable increase in alveolar pressure but does not contribute to the inspiratory threshold load or dynamic hyperinflation. Thus, precise measurement of auto-PEEP in spontaneously breathing patients may require monitoring of gastric pressure in addition to esophageal pressure. Whether precise quantification of auto-PEEP with the use of esophageal

and gastric pressure measurements results in better outcomes than qualitative detection of auto-PEEP through physical assessment is presently unknown [72].

Weaning from mechanical ventilation

Both volume and pressure loads are placed on the respiratory muscles in the patient with respiratory failure [73]. Using an esophageal balloon, the pressure loads can be expressed several ways. The pressure loads from the chest wall can be determined by measuring chest wall compliance, as discussed above. A direct measurement of the pressure loads on the respiratory muscles can be made during a spontaneous breath, which can be expressed as the work of breathing (WoB = $\int P_{eso} dV$) or the pressure time product (PTP = $\int P_{eso} dt$). The respiratory muscle pressure component of load is most closely correlated with respiratory muscle oxygen consumption [74,75]. PTP thus more closely correlates with oxygen demands and fatigue than work of breathing. Normal work of breathing per breath is 0.3 J/L to 0.7 J/L or 4 J to 8 J per minute. Normal PTP is 100 $H_2O \times sec \times min^{-1}$. It makes physiologic sense that discontinuation of mechanical ventilation will be unlikely if WoB or PTP is increased [76,77]. However, a threshold for either WoB or PTP that separates weaning success from failure has not been reported. Jubran and colleagues [78] reported that a trend index that quantified esophageal pressure swings during a spontaneous breathing trial provided additional guidance in patient management over tests used to decide

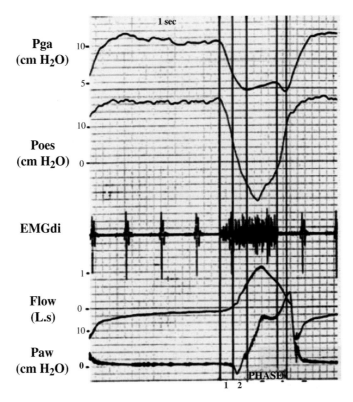

Fig. 8. Use of esophageal manometry to detect intrinsic PEEP. The figure shows a single assisted breath, with data displayed from a gastric manometer, esophageal manometer, EMG recorder of the diaphragm, and with flow and pressure measured at the airway. In phase 1 of breathing, esophageal pressure falls and the diaphragm is activated, yet no pressure change or positive flow is generated. Only after a certain threshold pressure is reached is flow initiated during phase 2. The pressure required to initiate flow is the amount of auto-PEEP. *Abbreviations:* P_{aw}, airway pressure; P_{ga}, gastric pressure. (*From* Brochard L. Intrinsic (or auto-) positive end-expiratory pressure during spontaneous or assisted ventilation. Intensive Care Med 2002;28(11):1552–4; with permission.)

when to initiate weaning. The advantage of the trend index may be related to the progressive increase in esophageal pressure throughout a failed weaning trial, whereas the more easily observed breathing pattern changed little after 2 minutes of spontaneous breathing. Although this approach is intriguing, the trend index requires a nonlinear model (multivariate adaptive regression spline or MARS analysis) that cannot be easily applied at the bedside.

Measurement and technical difficulties

Esophageal manometry is not an automated procedure; experience is needed to ensure accurate balloon placement and to interpret results. In the study by Talmor [70], measurements required 30 minutes and two to three investigators. Moreover,

the balloon-tipped catheters and associated monitoring equipment are not commonly available for clinical use.

Does the esophageal pressure accurately estimate pleural pressure?

There has been debate as to whether esophageal balloons accurately represent pleural pressure, particularly in the mechanically ventilated patient [79]. A number of assumptions must be made, including that the transmural esophageal pressure is negligible and that there is no compression of the esophagus by other intrathoracic structures (heart and mediastinum). These measurements are most easily made in awake, cooperative patients who can perform maneuvers to help confirm optimal balloon placement. Unfortunately, direct measurement is invasive, so comparison with a gold standard is difficult. Some of these concerns have been addressed. For example, Washko and colleagues [80] evaluated esophageal pressures in healthy subjects in both the sitting and supine position. There was a small change, partly explained by changes in relaxation volume (FRC) in the two positions, and partly by the change in position. The magnitude of change was less than 3 cm H_2O. Baydur and colleagues [81] also evaluated esophageal manometry at a variety of lung volumes and balloon positions within the esophagus; there were only small changes. However, it may not be valid to extrapolate data from normal subjects to that of critically ill mechanically ventilated patients.

While esophageal manometry is the standard method of estimating pleural pressure, pleural pressure changes during lung inflation are also transmitted to other structures in the mediastinum. In 1965, Comroe [82] suggested that an intrathoracic vein with its thin wall is capable of transmitting pleural pressure and might therefore be an acceptable alternative to the esophagus for pleural pressure measurement. In healthy adults, it has been shown that valid measurements of pleural pressure changes can be obtained from esophageal pressure or respiratory variation in central venous pressure [83]. In one study, it was suggested that respiratory variation in central venous pressure was more reliable than esophageal pressure in reflecting a change in pleural pressure in anesthetized supine patients [84]. Respiratory variation in central venous pressure is easily detected at the bedside during mechanical ventilation, and varies from a positive deflection when the respiratory muscles are completely inactive to negative swings during large inspiratory efforts. Chieveley-Williams and colleagues [85] recently compared changes in esophageal pressure to changes in central venous pressure and reported that useful information can be obtained from the respiratory variation in central venous pressure during mechanical ventilation.

Conclusion

While measurement of esophageal pressure during mechanical ventilation is theoretically appealing to measure the above parameters, no clinical trial has yet shown an outcome benefit of routine esophageal manometry in patients with acute respiratory failure.

Summary

Significant work remains to be done to tailor mechanical ventilation for individual patients. Exhaled breath condensate has potential as a marker for lung injury; however, further work is required before its use even in clinical trials. Pressure-volume curves and esophageal manometry have both been used in clinical trials, but our understanding of how best to employ the data derived from both is currently limited. Data for widespread use is currently lacking. Esophageal manometry in particular, however, may have a role in investigating failure to wean from mechanical ventilation. One marker of lung mechanics with some promise is the stress index; however, larger clinical trials are needed to confirm preliminary results.

References

[1] Slutsky AS, Tremblay LN. Multiple system organ failure. Is mechanical ventilation a contributing factor? Am J Respir Crit Care Med 1998;157(6 Pt 1): 1721–5.
[2] Ramnath VR, Hess DR, Thompson BT. Conventional mechanical ventilation in acute lung injury and acute respiratory distress syndrome. Clin Chest Med 2006;27(4):601–13, abstract viii.
[3] Terragni PP, Rosboch G, Tealdi A, et al. Tidal hyperinflation during low tidal volume ventilation in acute respiratory distress syndrome. Am J Respir Crit Care Med 2007;175(2):160–6.
[4] Brower RG, Lanken PN, MacIntyre N, et al. Higher versus lower positive end-expiratory pressures in patients with the acute respiratory distress syndrome. N Engl J Med 2004;351(4):327–36.
[5] Silkoff PE, Erzurum SC, Lundberg JO, et al. ATS workshop proceedings: exhaled nitric oxide and nitric oxide oxidative metabolism in exhaled breath condensate. Proc Am Thorac Soc 2006;3(2): 131–45.
[6] Jackson AS, Sandrini A, Campbell C, et al. Comparison of biomarkers in exhaled breath condensate and bronchoalveolar lavage. Am J Respir Crit Care Med 2007;175(3):222–7.
[7] Moloney ED, Mumby SE, Gajdocsi R, et al. Exhaled breath condensate detects markers of pulmonary inflammation after cardiothoracic surgery. Am J Respir Crit Care Med 2004;169(1):64–9.
[8] Soyer OU, Dizdar EA, Keskin O, et al. Comparison of two methods for exhaled breath condensate collection. Allergy 2006;61(8):1016–8.
[9] Prieto L, Ferrer A, Palop J, et al. Differences in exhaled breath condensate pH measurements between samples obtained with two commercial devices. Respir Med 2007;101(8):1715–20.

[10] Bloemen K, Lissens G, Desager K, et al. Determinants of variability of protein content, volume and pH of exhaled breath condensate. Respir Med 2007;101(6):1331–7.

[11] McCafferty JB, Bradshaw TA, Tate S, et al. Effects of breathing pattern and inspired air conditions on breath condensate volume, pH, nitrite, and protein concentrations. Thorax 2004;59(8):694–8.

[12] Baraldi E, Ghiro L, Piovan V, et al. Safety and success of exhaled breath condensate collection in asthma. Arch Dis Child 2003;88(4):358–60.

[13] Carpenter CT, Price PV, Christman BW. Exhaled breath condensate isoprostanes are elevated in patients with acute lung injury or ARDS. Chest 1998;114(6):1653–9.

[14] Balbi B, Pignatti P, Corradi M, et al. Bronchoalveolar lavage, sputum and exhaled clinically relevant inflammatory markers: values in healthy adults. Eur Respir J 2007;30(4):769–81.

[15] Paget-Brown AO, Ngamtrakulpanit L, Smith A, et al. Normative data for pH of exhaled breath condensate. Chest 2006;129(2):426–30.

[16] Corradi M, Pesci A, Casana R, et al. Nitrate in exhaled breath condensate of patients with different airway diseases. Nitric Oxide 2003;8(1):26–30.

[17] Gessner C, Hammerschmidt S, Kuhn H, et al. Breath condensate nitrite correlates with hyperinflation in chronic obstructive pulmonary disease. Respir Med 2007;101(11):2271–8.

[18] Gessner C, Hammerschmidt S, Kuhn H, et al. Exhaled breath condensate nitrite and its relation to tidal volume in acute lung injury. Chest 2003;124(3):1046–52.

[19] Hunt JF, Fang K, Malik R, et al. Endogenous airway acidification. Implications for asthma pathophysiology. Am J Respir Crit Care Med 2000;161(3 Pt 1):694–9.

[20] Kostikas K, Papatheodorou G, Ganas K, et al. pH in expired breath condensate of patients with inflammatory airway diseases. Am J Respir Crit Care Med 2002;165(10):1364–70.

[21] Gessner C, Hammerschmidt S, Kuhn H, et al. Exhaled breath condensate acidification in acute lung injury. Respir Med 2003;97(11):1188–94.

[22] Ricciardolo FL, Rado V, Fabbri LM, et al. Bronchoconstriction induced by citric acid inhalation in guinea pigs: role of tachykinins, bradykinin, and nitric oxide. Am J Respir Crit Care Med 1999;159(2):557–62.

[23] Luk CK, Dulfano MJ. Effect of pH, viscosity and ionic-strength changes on ciliary beating frequency of human bronchial explants. Clin Sci (Lond) 1983;64(4):449–51.

[24] Holma B, Lindegren M, Andersen JM. pH effects on ciliomotility and morphology of respiratory mucosa. Arch Environ Health 1977;32(5):216–26.

[25] Holma B, Hegg PO. pH- and protein-dependent buffer capacity and viscosity of respiratory mucus.

Their interrelationships and influence on health. Sci Total Environ 1989;84:71–82.

[26] Walsh BK, Mackey DJ, Pajewski T, et al. Exhaled-breath condensate pH can be safely and continuously monitored in mechanically ventilated patients. Respir Care 2006;51(10):1125–31.

[27] Carpagnano GE, Foschino Barbaro MP, Resta O, et al. Exhaled markers in the monitoring of airways inflammation and its response to steroid's treatment in mild persistent asthma. Eur J Pharmacol 2005;519(1–2):175–81.

[28] Biernacki WA, Kharitonov SA, Barnes PJ. Increased leukotriene B4 and 8-isoprostane in exhaled breath condensate of patients with exacerbations of COPD. Thorax 2003;58(4):294–8.

[29] Majewska E, Kasielski M, Luczynski R, et al. Elevated exhalation of hydrogen peroxide and thiobarbituric acid reactive substances in patients with community acquired pneumonia. Respir Med 2004;98(7):669–76.

[30] Fireman E, Shtark M, Priel IE, et al. Hydrogen peroxide in exhaled breath condensate (EBC) vs eosinophil count in induced sputum (IS) in parenchymal vs airways lung diseases. Inflammation 2007;30(1–2):44–51.

[31] Baldwin SR, Simon RH, Grum CM, et al. Oxidant activity in expired breath of patients with adult respiratory distress syndrome. Lancet 1986;1(8471):11–4.

[32] Sznajder JI, Fraiman A, Hall JB, et al. Increased hydrogen peroxide in the expired breath of patients with acute hypoxemic respiratory failure. Chest 1989;96(3):606–12.

[33] Bone RC. Diagnosis of causes for acute respiratory distress by pressure-volume curves. Chest 1976;70(6):740–6.

[34] Matamis D, Lemaire F, Harf A, et al. Total respiratory pressure-volume curves in the adult respiratory distress syndrome. Chest 1984;86(1):58–66.

[35] Suter PM, Fairley B, Isenberg MD. Optimum end-expiratory airway pressure in patients with acute pulmonary failure. N Engl J Med 1975;292(6):284–9.

[36] Dall'ava-Santucci J, Armaganidis A, Brunet F, et al. Mechanical effects of PEEP in patients with adult respiratory distress syndrome. J Appl Physiol 1990;68(3):843–8.

[37] Amato MB, Barbas CS, Medeiros DM, et al. Effect of a protective-ventilation strategy on mortality in the acute respiratory distress syndrome. N Engl J Med 1998;338(6):347–54.

[38] Ranieri VM, Suter PM, Tortorella C, et al. Effect of mechanical ventilation on inflammatory mediators in patients with acute respiratory distress syndrome: a randomized controlled trial. JAMA 1999;282(1):54–61.

[39] Villar J, Kacmarek RM, Perez-Mendez L, et al. A high positive end-expiratory pressure, low tidal volume ventilatory strategy improves outcome in

persistent acute respiratory distress syndrome: a randomized, controlled trial. Crit Care Med 2006;34(5): 1311–8.

[40] Hickling KG. The pressure-volume curve is greatly modified by recruitment. A mathematical model of ARDS lungs. Am J Respir Crit Care Med 1998; 158(1):194–202.

[41] Jonson B, Richard JC, Straus C, et al. Pressure-volume curves and compliance in acute lung injury: evidence of recruitment above the lower inflection point. Am J Respir Crit Care Med 1999;159(4 Pt 1):1172–8.

[42] Albaiceta GM, Taboada F, Parra D, et al. Tomographic study of the inflection points of the pressure-volume curve in acute lung injury. Am J Respir Crit Care Med 2004;170(10):1066–72.

[43] Schiller HJ, Steinberg J, Halter J, et al. Alveolar inflation during generation of a quasi-static pressure/volume curve in the acutely injured lung. Crit Care Med 2003;31(4):1126–33.

[44] Mergoni M, Martelli A, Olpi A, et al. Impact of positive end-expiratory pressure on chest wall and lung pressure-volume curve in acute respiratory failure. Am J Respir Crit Care Med 1997;156(3 Pt 1):846–54.

[45] Ranieri VM, Brienza N, Santostasi S, et al. Impairment of lung and chest wall mechanics in patients with acute respiratory distress syndrome: role of abdominal distension. Am J Respir Crit Care Med 1997;156(4 Pt 1):1082–91.

[46] Hickling KG. Best compliance during a decremental, but not incremental, positive end-expiratory pressure trial is related to open-lung positive end-expiratory pressure: a mathematical model of acute respiratory distress syndrome lungs. Am J Respir Crit Care Med 2001;163(1):69–78.

[47] Holzapfel L, Robert D, Perrin F, et al. Static pressure-volume curves and effect of positive end-expiratory pressure on gas exchange in adult respiratory distress syndrome. Crit Care Med 1983;11(8):591–7.

[48] Rimensberger PC, Pristine G, Mullen BM, et al. Lung recruitment during small tidal volume ventilation allows minimal positive end-expiratory pressure without augmenting lung injury. Crit Care Med 1999;27(9):1940–5.

[49] Rimensberger PC, Cox PN, Frndova H, et al. The open lung during small tidal volume ventilation: concepts of recruitment and "optimal" positive end-expiratory pressure. Crit Care Med 1999;27(9): 1946–52.

[50] Bindslev L, Hedenstierna G, Santesson J, et al. Airway closure during anaesthesia, and its prevention by positive end expiratory pressure. Acta Anaesthesiol Scand 1980;24(3):199–205.

[51] Salmon RB, Primiano FP Jr, Saidel GM, et al. Human lung pressure-volume relationships: alveolar collapse and airway closure. J Appl Physiol 1981; 51(2):353–62.

[52] Albaiceta GM, Luyando LH, Parra D, et al. Inspiratory vs. expiratory pressure-volume curves to set end-expiratory pressure in acute lung injury. Intensive Care Med 2005;31(10):1370–8.

[53] Dall'ava-Santucci J, Armaganidis A, Brunet F, et al. Causes of error of respiratory pressure-volume curves in paralyzed subjects. J Appl Physiol 1988; 64(1):42–9.

[54] Decailliot F, Demoule A, Maggiore SM, et al. Pressure-volume curves with and without muscle paralysis in acute respiratory distress syndrome. Intensive Care Med 2006;32(9):1322–8.

[55] Lee WL, Stewart TE, MacDonald R, et al. Safety of pressure-volume curve measurement in acute lung injury and ARDS using a syringe technique. Chest 2002;121(5):1595–601.

[56] Roch A, Forel JM, Demory D, et al. Generation of a single pulmonary pressure-volume curve does not durably affect oxygenation in patients with acute respiratory distress syndrome. Crit Care 2006;10(3): R85.

[57] Harris RS. Pressure-volume curves of the respiratory system. Respir Care 2005;50(1):78–98 [discussion: 98–9].

[58] Karason S, Sondergaard S, Lundin S, et al. A new method for non-invasive, manoeuvre-free determination of "static" pressure-volume curves during dynamic/therapeutic mechanical ventilation. Acta Anaesthesiol Scand 2000;44(5):578–85.

[59] Karason S, Sondergaard S, Lundin S, et al. Continuous on-line measurements of respiratory system, lung and chest wall mechanics during mechanic ventilation. Intensive Care Med 2001;27(8): 1328–39.

[60] Karason S, Sondergaard S, Lundin S, et al. Direct tracheal airway pressure measurements are essential for safe and accurate dynamic monitoring of respiratory mechanics. A laboratory study. Acta Anaesthesiol Scand 2001;45(2):173–9.

[61] Sondergaard S, Karason S, Wiklund J, et al. Alveolar pressure monitoring: an evaluation in a lung model and in patients with acute lung injury. Intensive Care Med 2003;29(6):955–62.

[62] Karason S, Sondergaard S, Lundin S, et al. Evaluation of pressure/volume loops based on intratracheal pressure measurements during dynamic conditions. Acta Anaesthesiol Scand 2000;44(5): 571–7.

[63] Adams AB, Cakar N, Marini JJ. Static and dynamic pressure-volume curves reflect different aspects of respiratory system mechanics in experimental acute respiratory distress syndrome. Respir Care 2001; 46(7):686–93.

[64] Stahl CA, Moller K, Schumann S, et al. Dynamic versus static respiratory mechanics in acute lung injury and acute respiratory distress syndrome. Crit Care Med 2006;34(8):2090–8.

[65] Harris RS, Hess DR, Venegas JG. An objective analysis of the pressure-volume curve in the acute respiratory distress syndrome. Am J Respir Crit Care Med 2000;161(2 Pt 1):432–9.

[66] Venegas JG, Harris RS, Simon BA. A comprehensive equation for the pulmonary pressure-volume curve. J Appl Physiol 1998;84(1):389–95.

[67] Ranieri VM, Zhang H, Mascia L, et al. Pressure-time curve predicts minimally injurious ventilatory strategy in an isolated rat lung model. Anesthesiology 2000;93(5):1320–8.

[68] Grasso S, Terragni P, Mascia L, et al. Airway pressure-time curve profile (stress index) detects tidal recruitment/hyperinflation in experimental acute lung injury. Crit Care Med 2004;32(4):1018–27.

[69] Grasso S, Stripoli T, De Michele M, et al. ARDSnet ventilatory protocol and alveolar hyperinflation: role of positive end-expiratory pressure. Am J Respir Crit Care Med 2007;176(8):761–7.

[70] Talmor D, Sarge T, O'Donnell CR, et al. Esophageal and transpulmonary pressures in acute respiratory failure. Crit Care Med 2006;34(5):1389–94.

[71] Brochard L. Intrinsic (or auto-) positive end-expiratory pressure during spontaneous or assisted ventilation. Intensive Care Med 2002;28(11):1552–4.

[72] Kress JP, O'Connor MF, Schmidt GA. Clinical examination reliably detects intrinsic positive end-expiratory pressure in critically ill, mechanically ventilated patients. Am J Respir Crit Care Med 1999; 159(1):290–4.

[73] MacIntyre NR. Respiratory mechanics in the patient who is weaning from the ventilator. Respir Care 2005;50(2):275–86 [discussion: 284–6].

[74] MacIntyre NR, Leatherman NE. Mechanical loads on the ventilatory muscles. A theoretical analysis. Am Rev Respir Dis 1989;139(4):968–73.

[75] McGregor M, Becklake MR. The relationship of oxygen cost of breathing to respiratory mechanical work and respiratory force. J Clin Invest 1961;40:971–80.

[76] Fiastro JF, Habib MP, Shon BY, et al. Comparison of standard weaning parameters and the mechanical work of breathing in mechanically ventilated patients. Chest 1988;94(2):232–8.

[77] Jubran A, Tobin MJ. Pathophysiologic basis of acute respiratory distress in patients who fail a trial of weaning from mechanical ventilation. Am J Respir Crit Care Med 1997;155(3):906–15.

[78] Jubran A, Grant BJ, Laghi F, et al. Weaning prediction: esophageal pressure monitoring complements readiness testing. Am J Respir Crit Care Med 2005;171(11):1252–9.

[79] Hager DN, Brower RG. Customizing lung-protective mechanical ventilation strategies. Crit Care Med 2006;34(5):1554–5.

[80] Washko GR, O'Donnell CR, Loring SH. Volume-related and volume-independent effects of posture on esophageal and transpulmonary pressures in healthy subjects. J Appl Physiol 2006;100(3): 753–8.

[81] Baydur A, Cha EJ, Sassoon CS. Validation of esophageal balloon technique at different lung volumes and postures. J Appl Physiol 1987;62(1): 315–21.

[82] Comroe J. Physiology of respiration. Chicago: Year Book Medical Publishers; 1965.

[83] Flemale A, Gillard C, Dierckx JP. Comparison of central venous, oesophageal and mouth occlusion pressure with water-filled catheters for estimating pleural pressure changes in healthy adults. Eur Respir J 1988;1(1):51–7.

[84] Walling PT, Savege TM. A comparison of oesophageal and central venous pressures in the measurement of transpulmonary pressure change. Br J Anaesth 1976;48(5):475–9.

[85] Chieveley-Williams S, Dinner L, Puddicombe A, et al. Central venous and bladder pressure reflect transdiaphragmatic pressure during pressure support ventilation. Chest 2002;121(2):533–8.

ELSEVIER
SAUNDERS

Clin Chest Med 29 (2008) 313–321

CLINICS
IN CHEST
MEDICINE

Effects of Respiratory-Therapist Driven Protocols on House-Staff Knowledge and Education of Mechanical Ventilation

Jessica Y. Chia, MD[a],*, Alison S. Clay, MD[b]

[a]Department of Medicine, Division of Pulmonary and Critical Care Medicine, Duke University Medical Center, Box 2634, Durham, NC 27710, USA
[b]Departments of Surgery and Medicine, Duke University Medical Center, Box 2945, Durham, NC 27710, USA

The intensive care unit (ICU) is a place of high-acuity illness with inherently high morbidity, enormous cost and resource use, and traditionally, high practice variability, with major variation in accepted clinical practices [1,2]. Those in academic medical centers are no exception, with idiosyncratic practice patterns often guided more by local opinion and supply of resources than by science [3]. Unnecessary variation in clinical care increases the likelihood of errors and contributes to the high cost of ICU care. The large numbers of house-staff in academic medical centers who provide most of the front-line care and decision-making, may augment this high practice variability and potential for medical errors. This article discusses strategies to minimize practice variability through the implementation of guidelines and protocols, difficulties with and barriers to the effective use of these decision-support systems, means to overcome these barriers, and the impact of this entire process on house-staff education.

Precisely because of the nature of critical care medicine, replete with high morbidity, cost, and practice variation, considerable interest has been devoted to attempts at standardizing patient care, with the hopes of improving care delivery, patient outcomes, and resource use. Several large, randomized, prospective clinical trials have shown that protocol-based strategies can reduce variation and cost of ICU medicine, increase adherence to evidence-based interventions, and reduce error, thereby improving morbidity and mortality of

critically ill patients [4–7]. Areas in which ICU protocols have been successful in improving patient outcomes include sedation and neuromuscular blockade use, and ventilator management [4,7–9].

Mechanical ventilation is one of the most common ICU therapies and one that is associated with tremendous risk and cost. These include increased mortality, nosocomial and ventilator-associated pneumonia, ventilator-associated lung injury, airway trauma, and increased need for sedation [10–12]. Use of the ventilator for more than 21 days is associated with costs exceeding $400,000, and patients who require prolonged mechanical ventilation often suffer from posttraumatic stress disorder and decreased indices on social functioning scales [13]. Despite this, studies have shown that patients are kept on the ventilator too long: of the patients screened for enrollment in two ventilator weaning studies, more than 70% were considered candidates for immediate extubation [14,15]. On the other hand, premature discontinuation of mechanical ventilation and extubation failure is also associated with considerable morbidity, mortality, and costs [16–18]. To avoid these pitfalls, evidence-based mechanical ventilation guidelines and protocols have been developed to assist clinicians in managing patients who require mechanical ventilation [19–22]. The consensus report of a task force convened by the Society of Critical Care Medicine leadership to ascertain a "best" practice model of ICU critical care delivery highlighted, among other things, the use of standards, protocols, and guidelines to assure consistent approaches to medical, nursing, and technical issues [23].

* Corresponding author.
E-mail address: chia0002@mc.duke.edu (J.Y. Chia).

Merits and perils of guidelines and protocols

Despite the development of guidelines and protocols by experts, their implementation in medicine has not been without controversy. Guidelines and their very specific applications, in the form of protocols and algorithms, have been a subject of great debate since their burgeoning popularity in the last two decades [24]. Understanding this controversy requires an appreciation of the difference between guidelines and protocols. Guidelines, defined as general statements that lack detail and provide broad guidance that requires clinicians to fill in gaps with their own judgment, background, and experience, allow different decisions by different clinicians for the same clinical scenario. In contrast, protocols are detailed, "adequately explicit" rules for decision-making based on individual patient data, thereby generating patient-specific therapy instructions that can be performed by different clinicians with almost no interclinician variability [6,25].

Both of these decision-support systems have evolved as strategies to standardize care, principally by reducing practice variability. They must be based on sound evidence, supplemented where necessary by truly expert opinion; they represent a desire to assure quality care and to guarantee some degree of consistency from patient to patient; and when properly implemented, they offer a means for providing patients with a minimum level of standardized care [8,24–26]. They provide a link between theory and practice, promoting "best practice" from "best evidence," improving efficiency and uniformity of care, reducing error rates, and promoting collaboration and a multidisciplinary approach among care providers. In doing so, they have favorable effects on clinician and patient outcomes in the ICU [5,7,8,25]. They are often viewed as safeguards to ensure that certain practices and procedures are performed expeditiously, and as a mechanism to implement evidence-based medicine with the primary goal of providing the best possible care, with subsequent cost reduction and efficiency improvement as a result of implementing the best medical practice [8]. The evidence that guidelines and explicit decision-support systems improve health care outcomes is consistent with results from systems approaches in other fields [5]. System stabilization through reduction in practice variation is a prerequisite for continuous quality improvement, and this is a central theme in the application of the Six Sigma methodology to health care [6].

To counter these views, critics of guidelines and protocols argue that evidence-based medicine can be practiced without the use of protocols, and raise valid concerns that they promote a "cookbook medicine" approach that restricts analytic and critical thought, clinical innovation, and individualized care. The removal of thought and judgment from clinical decision-making leads to a dulling of critical thinking and de-skilling, breeds complacency, and stifles learning. Protocols can be inflexible, too rigid, and challenge physician autonomy. There is concern that third parties, potentially influenced by financial or legal incentives, may use guidelines to curtail treatment choice [27], or may use them with punitive intent and in litigation. Additionally, and perhaps more relevant, the introduction of guidelines and protocols into an institution or ICU does not guarantee that they will be used, or used properly. Protocols do not assure good care, especially if incorrectly applied.

Compliance with guidelines and effective use of protocols (or not?)

The controversies surrounding the use of guidelines and protocols are manifested, perhaps, by the poor adherence to and limited impact of practice guidelines. Few guidelines lead to consistent changes in provider behavior, and most have only modest and limited impact [28,29]. Studies show that physicians are often noncompliant with guidelines and other decision-support systems, as seen in the persistently low adherence rates reported for the National Asthma Education and Prevention Program Expert Panel's Guidelines for the Diagnosis and Management of Asthma [30]. In a national survey of United States pediatricians, where 88% expressed familiarity with asthma guidelines, only 35% actually followed guidelines [31]. The overall lack of behavioral effects from clinical practice guidelines is not limited to asthma diagnosis and treatment, either in pulmonary medicine or in other fields [32,33]. One meta-analysis found that the mean compliance to clinical recommendations across a variety of medical conditions was only 54.4% [34].

This is also true in the case of mechanical ventilation. Variation in ICU practices and clinical management is associated with differences in patient outcomes and increased costs [7,8], and mechanical ventilation protocols improve outcomes over ad hoc or "usual care" decisions made by clinicians [22,35–41]. Yet despite having official guidelines and standardized procedures in place, compliance is notoriously low [42–44]. In one randomized, controlled trial of weaning protocols in pediatric patients, adherence was 66% [45]. In the weaning protocol implementation study by Ely and colleagues [46], intensive physician and nonphysician education and feedback were used to promote protocol adherence, but despite those efforts, adherence was only 25% to 36% over the final 6 months of implementation. Perhaps most telling is the behavior of the National Institutes of Health Acute Respiratory Distress Syndrome (ARDS) Network, an accepted group of experts who demonstrated clearly in 2000 that tidal volumes in ARDS patients of 6 mL/kg (ideal body weight) produced better survival than the traditional 12 mL/kg tidal volume in widespread use at the time [47]. Despite this, the next two trials conducted by this group in 2004 and 2006 reported prerandomization tidal volumes (ie, tidal volumes being used by clinicians in their institutions before entering the trial) still above this target: 8.1 mL/kg and 7.4 mL/kg (ideal body weight), respectively [48,49].

Studies to address why physicians are so poor at following guidelines and protocols have found various barriers to adherence, including: lack of awareness, familiarity, or agreement with the protocol; lack of self-efficacy or expectations about outcomes; the inertia of previous practices; and external barriers (guideline-, patient-, and environment-related), such as guidelines being inconvenient, cumbersome, confusing, or difficult to use [27,50].

In an attempt to circumvent these barriers to the effective use of protocols, some have implemented physician-independent treatment algorithms run by nurses and respiratory therapists. Current evidence suggests that respiratory therapist-driven protocols for ventilator management and weaning results in shorter duration of mechanical ventilation compared with traditional physician-directed weaning, reduced costs, and improved resource allocation [36–39,41,46,51–59]. In one study, respiratory therapist-driven protocols in patients requiring prolonged mechanical ventilation reduced median weaning time by almost 12 days [60].

The superior outcomes obtained with nonphysician run protocols for mechanical ventilation has led a collective task force of pulmonary and critical care experts, facilitated by the American College of Chest Physicians (ACCP), the American Association for Respiratory Care, and the American College of Critical Care Medicine, to recommend that ICUs develop and implement respiratory-care protocols designed for nonphysician health care professionals [19,22].

The effect of protocols on house-staff education

If we can agree that mechanical ventilation protocols are best for patient care and are more successful when run by respiratory therapists, how are house-staff (who have effectively been removed from the feedback loop) going to learn the principles of mechanical ventilation?

This question is particularly sobering when one considers the current state of trainee knowledge in mechanical ventilation. In 2003, Cox and colleagues [61] conducted a nationwide study assessing the knowledge of 259 senior internal medicine residents at the completion of their residency. They found that only 52% could identify the appropriate tidal volume for a patient with ARDS, 38% could not recognize patients who were ready for weaning trials, and nearly one-third could not recognize indications for noninvasive ventilation. This is significant because all three concepts (low tidal volume ventilation in ARDS, daily awakenings and spontaneous breathing trials, and appropriate use of noninvasive positive pressure ventilation) have been associated with lower mortality and reduced health care costs [36,47,62]. Another alarming finding in Cox's study was that almost 50% of the surveyed residents felt dissatisfied with their training in mechanical ventilation, and many felt that what they did know was barely adequate for providing effective patient care [61].

Do protocols contribute to this knowledge deficit or are protocols the solution to it?

Explicit decision-support instruments such as protocols can be effective teaching tools. Provided that protocols are rigorously reviewed and evidence-based, they promote quality and standardization of care. They also specify the important variables to be considered and the rules for using them to make decisions. For house-staff moving between day and night shifts, and between supervising fellows and attendings, the consistent application of rules for mechanical ventilation may promote mastery of medical knowledge specific to mechanical ventilation. If trainees are able to explain the rationale for the decisions guided by protocols, they demonstrate patient care competence. If protocols are seen as works in progress that require continual review and revision through the appropriate collection of data, then trainees demonstrate practice-based learning and improvements in systems-based practice.

On the other hand, by limiting practice variation (and potentially certain modes of ventilation) through the use of mechanical ventilation protocols, trainees may not be able to apply their knowledge to difficult circumstances, may not know when to break from protocol or how to manage a patient outside of protocol, and may not cope well or easily adapt to circumstances in other institutions where ventilator protocols are either used differently or not used at all.

The Duke experience: what do we know about how residents learn in an environment where protocols are used?

At Duke University Medical Center (DUMC), respiratory-therapist driven protocols have been used since 1996 to limit tidal volumes to 5 mL/kg to 7 mL/kg in all patients, regardless of diagnosis, using predominately pressure modes of ventilation. This protocol is used in DUMC's surgery/ trauma, neurology, cardiology, and medical ICUs. Third and fourth quarter evaluation of 206 patients (January to June, 2007) receiving high level assist-control or pressure support modes of ventilation for respiratory failure, had an average tidal volume of 7.3 mL/kg (ideal body weight). Interestingly, the largest tidal volumes were seen in those receiving low levels of support in the recovering and weaning phase of their disease. Comparisons to others' data are difficult because most studies look only at patients with ARDS, but these values are generally lower than those published [44,63]. The DUMC's protocol also includes evaluation for and completion of a spontaneous breathing trial in eligible patients. Of 374 patients evaluated in the third and fourth quarters this year, 137 were eligible for spontaneous breathing trials (SBT) and 89.8% of those actually had one completed, again with values better than those published [15].

In this environment, 46 second-year internal medicine residents were evaluated at the beginning and end of their 6-week medical ICU rotation on their self-confidence in various different domains of critical care medicine (Alison S. Clay, MD, personal communication, 2007). Three domains pertained to mechanical ventilation: use of mechanical ventilation to manage respiratory failure, use of respiratory mechanics to predict ventilator liberation, and application of noninvasive ventilation. At the start of the rotation, residents ranked themselves as less than competent in all three areas. At the end of the rotation, residents on average considered themselves at least competent (though not proficient) in the use of mechanical ventilation to manage respiratory failure, and demonstrated statistically significant improvements in self-confidence in all three domains during the rotation (Fig. 1), a finding consistent with that of Cox and colleagues [61] (Alison S. Clay, MD, personal communication, 2007).

Residents also completed a 45-question, knowledge-based, multiple-choice test, with 12 of the 45 questions related to the use of mechanical ventilation. Nine of those 12 questions were taken with permission from Cox's validated test, with the others taken from ACCP and American College of Physicians board review materials. At the start of the rotation, the mean score on those 12 questions on mechanical ventilation was 59%, and improved to 67% at the end of rotation ($P = .01$) (Alison S. Clay, MD, personal communication, 2007).

Direct comparisons to Cox's study are difficult because the Duke residents were all second year residents (compared with senior residents), had less than 2 months of ICU exposure, worked in a closed ICU at a single institution, and were just completing their rotation. Looking at the nine questions common to both Cox and the authors' experience, the DUMC second-year residents scored 64.5% at the start of rotation, and improved to 74.7% at the end of rotation ($P = .006$). Likewise, senior residents evaluated in Cox's study scored 74.7% on those nine questions. In regards to specific topics, 81% of DUMC residents following their ICU experience versus 73% of the national cohort of residents could identify the appropriate use of noninvasive ventilation ($P = .3$), and 81% of DUMC residents versus 62% of the national cohort of residents ($P = .02$) could identify the appropriate timing and need for an SBT [62] (Alison S. Clay, MD, personal communication, 2007).

This crudely shows that the average second-year medicine resident at the conclusion of his or her 6-week medical ICU rotation at an institution heavily reliant on respiratory therapist-driven mechanical ventilation protocols performed at least as well as the cohort studied by Cox. This also shows that house-staff knowledge of mechanical ventilation improved during the DUMC ICU

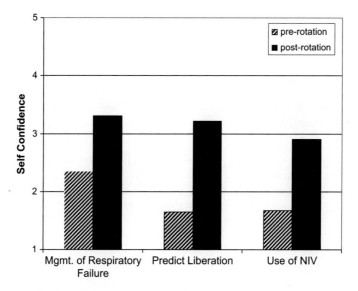

Fig. 1. Self-confidence of Duke University second year medicine residents regarding use of mechanical ventilation, pre- and postmedical ICU rotation. Self confidence rating scale: 1, novice; 2, advanced beginner; 3, competent; 4, proficient; 5, master. NIV, noninvasive ventilation.

rotation, in spite of (or perhaps, because of) a respiratory therapist-driven protocol. However, this still highlights the vast knowledge deficiency and the low self-confidence regarding the use of mechanical ventilation, and the definite need for improvement.

Protocols may be the answer, but this depends on the attitudes of learners and teachers toward them. To assess the attitudes of DUMC's learners and teachers toward mechanical ventilation protocols, and their perception of the protocols' effects on patient care and education, the authors surveyed a convenience sample of 175 physicians (internal medicine residents, pulmonary and critical care fellows, and pulmonary and critical care attendings), ICU nurses, and respiratory therapists at Duke University (Fig. 2). Each person was first asked if he or she had ever practiced

or trained at an institution that did not use mechanical ventilation protocols in their ICU. Respondents were then asked if they thought "ventilator protocols hindered patient care, or improved patient care" and if "ventilator protocols hindered teaching of mechanical ventilation principles to medical students and residents, or assisted teaching of mechanical ventilation principles to medical students and residents."

Approximately half of the respondents had only worked in ICUs that employed mechanical ventilation protocols; 51% had ICU experience both with and without the use of these protocols. Of the respondents, 96% felt that ventilator protocols improved patient care, but 61% felt the protocols had a negative impact on teaching. Those who had ICU experience both with and without the use of mechanical ventilation

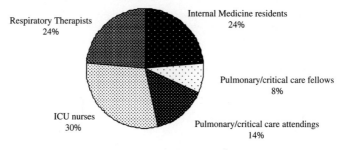

Fig. 2. Respondents to survey on attitudes toward mechanical ventilation protocols.

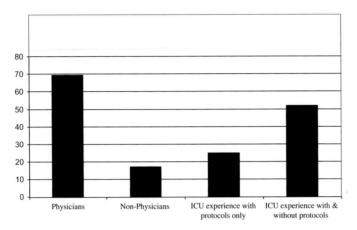

Fig. 3. Results of survey on attitudes toward mechanical ventilation protocols showing percentage of respondents who believe that protocols hinder teaching.

protocols were more likely to feel that protocols hindered teaching than those who only had experience in units with protocols (52% versus 25%, $P = .001$) (Fig. 3). Physicians were much more likely to believe that protocols impaired teaching than nonphysicians (68.8% versus 17.1%, $P < .001$). Although physicians were more likely to have ICU experience with and without the use of protocols, when analysis was limited to only those with both experiences, physicians were still more likely to believe that protocols hindered teaching than nonphysicians were (76.7% versus 23.4%, $P < .001$). Among physicians, fellows were more likely to view protocols as having a negative influence on education than either residents or faculty. The discrepancy in attitudes between physicians and nonphysicians, and between physicians with different levels of experience (residents, fellows, attendings) is likely related to the depth of understanding and level of competence expected from each.

It may be possible to synchronize our processes for improving patient care with our desire to improve medical education. The basic and most fundamental principle for our trainees is simply medical knowledge. Protocols allow us to introduce consistent principles of mechanical ventilation. Acquisition of this knowledge can be assessed with multiple-choice tests, which serve as a way to provide feedback to our trainees. When medical knowledge is not adequate, it can be improved with specific didactic sessions and online lectures (just as others have improved compliance with guidelines by increasing education of those guidelines). The application of protocols to individual patients requires a higher level of competence (the core

competency of patient care), which could be demonstrated at the bedside on rounds, through self-directed learning, or by rounding with respiratory therapists to demonstrate agility with actual use of protocols. Simulations would provide a higher stakes assessment of skill in patient care. Using quality improvement data that is already collected, or collecting new data from a unit, several units, or an institution, and critically analyzing that data to identify variations in practice or flagrant deviations from protocols, is the core competency of practice-based learning and improvement and is essentially feedback on practice (as opposed to feedback on knowledge). Understanding a system well enough to propose changes that further improve care is the highest-level competency, systems-based practice, and the perfect intersection of medical education and patient care.

Summary

In summary, it is clear that mechanical ventilator protocols in the ICU are best for patient care, decreasing patient time on the ventilator, and are often more successful when run by non-physicians. Moreover, because protocols employ evidence-based best practices to standardize care, protocols can be effective teaching tools, provided that trainees master the principles underlying the protocol and are able to explain the rationale for the decisions they make, implementing and applying the protocol with clinical acumen and with attention to individual subtleties [9]. Guidelines and protocols are neither panacea nor poison, just imperfect attempts to better care for patients. They should be viewed as dynamic tools in evolution that can provide a point of reference with which to compare and measure the need for current and future refinements. The real challenge, then, is to involve trainees in this process, commensurate with their level of experience and desired level of competence. "A well-designed ICU protocol does not constrain decision-making, but rather focuses a provider's attention on the common aspects of patients with a well-described illness. Protocol-driven care does not eliminate the need for clinical judgment. In fact, it demands constant attention to the subtleties inherent to each patient and may require deviations from the protocols. Protocol-driven care does not obviate the need for lifelong learning. On the contrary, it requires continual appraisal of evidence from the published literature so that protocols may be modified when new strategies of care have been demonstrated as effective and efficient" [9].

References

[1] Knaus WA, Wagner DP, Zimmerman JE, et al. Variations in mortality and length of stay in intensive care units. Ann Intern Med 1993;118(10): 753–61.

[2] Wennberg JE, Freeman JL, Shelton RM, et al. Hospital use and mortality among Medicare beneficiaries in Boston and New Haven. N Engl J Med 1989;321(17):1168–73.

[3] Wennberg JE. Unwarranted variations in healthcare delivery: implications for academic medical centres. BMJ 2002;325(7370):961–4.

[4] Holcomb BW, Wheeler AP, Ely EW. New ways to reduce unnecessary variation and improve outcomes in the intensive care unit. Curr Opin Crit Care 2001; 7(4):304–11.

[5] Morris AH. Decision support and safety of clinical environments. Qual Saf Health Care 2002;11(1): 69–75.

[6] Chatburn RL, Deem S. Respiratory controversies in the critical care setting. Should weaning protocols be used with all patients who receive mechanical ventilation? Respir Care 2007;52(5):609–19 [discussion: 619–21].

[7] Hammond JJ. Protocols and guidelines in critical care: development and implementation. Curr Opin Crit Care 2001;7(6):464–8.

[8] Ibrahim EH, Kollef MH. Using protocols to improve the outcomes of mechanically ventilated patients. Focus on weaning and sedation. Crit Care Clin 2001;17(4):989–1001.

[9] Wall RJ, Dittus RS, Ely EW. Protocol-driven care in the intensive care unit: a tool for quality. Crit Care 2001;5(6):283–5.

[10] Cook DJ, Walter SD, Cook RJ, et al. Incidence of and risk factors for ventilator-associated pneumonia in critically ill patients. Ann Intern Med 1998;129(6): 433–40.

[11] McLean SE, Jensen LA, Schroeder DG, et al. Improving adherence to a mechanical ventilation weaning protocol for critically ill adults: outcomes after an implementation program. Am J Crit Care 2006;15(3):299–309.

[12] Slutsky AS, Tremblay LN. Multiple system organ failure. Is mechanical ventilation a contributing factor? Am J Respir Crit Care Med 1998;157(6 Pt 1): 1721–5.

[13] Cox CE, Carson SS, Lindquist JH, et al. Differences in one-year health outcomes and resource utilization by definition of prolonged mechanical ventilation: a prospective cohort study. Crit Care 2007;11(1):R9.

[14] Brochard L, Rauss A, Benito S, et al. Comparison of three methods of gradual withdrawal from ventilatory support during weaning from mechanical ventilation. Am J Respir Crit Care Med 1994; 150(4):896–903.

[15] Esteban A, Frutos F, Tobin MJ, et al. A comparison of four methods of weaning patients from mechanical ventilation. Spanish Lung Failure Collaborative Group. N Engl J Med 1995;332(6):345–50.

[16] Epstein SK, Ciubotaru RL. Independent effects of etiology of failure and time to reintubation on outcome for patients failing extubation. Am J Respir Crit Care Med 1998;158(2):489–93.

[17] Epstein SK, Ciubotaru RL, Wong JB. Effect of failed extubation on the outcome of mechanical ventilation. Chest 1997;112(1):186–92.

[18] Esteban A, Alia I, Gordo F, et al. Extubation outcome after spontaneous breathing trials with T-tube or pressure support ventilation. The Spanish Lung Failure Collaborative Group. Am J Respir Crit Care Med 1997;156(2 Pt 1):459–65.

[19] MacIntyre NR, Cook DJ, Ely EW Jr, et al. Evidence-based guidelines for weaning and discontinuing ventilatory support: a collective task force facilitated by the American College of Chest Physicians; the American Association for Respiratory Care; and the American College of Critical Care Medicine. Chest 2001;120(6 Suppl):375S–95S.

[20] Pauwels RA, Buist AS, Calverley PM, et al. Global strategy for the diagnosis, management, and prevention of chronic obstructive pulmonary disease. NHLBI/WHO Global Initiative for Chronic Obstructive Lung Disease (GOLD) Workshop summary. Am J Respir Crit Care Med 2001;163(5): 1256–76.

[21] Brower RG, Ware LB, Berthiaume Y, et al. Treatment of ARDS. Chest 2001;120(4):1347–67.

[22] Ely EW, Meade MO, Haponik EF, et al. Mechanical ventilator weaning protocols driven by nonphysician health-care professionals: evidence-based clinical practice guidelines. Chest 2001;120(6 Suppl): 454S–63S.

[23] Brilli RJ, Spevetz A, Branson RD, et al. Critical care delivery in the intensive care unit: defining clinical roles and the best practice model. Crit Care Med 2001;29(10):2007–19.

[24] Dans PE. Credibility, cookbook medicine, and common sense: guidelines and the college. Ann Intern Med 1994;120(11):966–8.

[25] Morris AH. Treatment algorithms and protocolized care. Curr Opin Crit Care 2003;9(3):236–40.

[26] Woolf SH. Practice guidelines, a new reality in medicine. II. Methods of developing guidelines. Arch Intern Med 1992;152(5):946–52.

[27] Timmermans S, Mauck A. The promises and pitfalls of evidence-based medicine. Health Aff (Millwood) 2005;24(1):18–28.

[28] Redman BK. Clinical practice guidelines as tools of public policy: conflicts of purpose, issues of autonomy, and justice. J Clin Ethics 1994;5(4):303–9.

[29] Safran C, Rind DM, Davis RB, et al. Effects of a knowledge-based electronic patient record in adherence to practice guidelines. MD Comput 1996;13(1):55–63.

[30] Legorreta AP, Christian-Herman J, O'Connor RD, et al. Compliance with National Asthma Management Guidelines and specialty care: a health maintenance organization experience. Arch Intern Med 1998;158(5):457–64.

[31] Flores G, Lee M, Bauchner H, et al. Pediatricians' attitudes, beliefs, and practices regarding clinical practice guidelines: a national survey. Pediatrics 2000;105(3 Pt 1):496–501.

[32] Armstrong D. Clinical autonomy, individual and collective: the problem of changing doctors' behaviour. Soc Sci Med 2002;55(10):1771–7.

[33] Tapson VF, Decousus H, Pini M, et al. Venous thromboembolism prophylaxis in acutely ill hospitalized medical patients: findings from the International Medical Prevention Registry on Venous Thromboembolism. Chest 2007;132(3):936–45.

[34] Grilli R, Lomas J. Evaluating the message: the relationship between compliance rate and the subject of a practice guideline. Med Care 1994;32(3):202–13.

[35] Cohen IL, Bari N, Strosberg MA, et al. Reduction of duration and cost of mechanical ventilation in an intensive care unit by use of a ventilatory management team. Crit Care Med 1991;19(10):1278–84.

[36] Ely EW, Baker AM, Dunagan DP, et al. Effect on the duration of mechanical ventilation of identifying patients capable of breathing spontaneously. N Engl J Med 1996;335(25):1864–9.

[37] Epstein SK. Weaning from mechanical ventilation. Respir Care 2002;47(4):454–66 [discussion: 466–8].

[38] Horst HM, Mouro D, Hall-Jenssens RA, et al. Decrease in ventilation time with a standardized weaning process. Arch Surg 1998;133(5):483–8 [discussion: 488–9].

[39] Meade MO, Guyatt GH, Cook DJ. Weaning from mechanical ventilation: the evidence from clinical research. Respir Care 2001;46(12):1408–15 [discussion: 1415–7].

[40] Saura P, Blanch L, Mestre J, et al. Clinical consequences of the implementation of a weaning protocol. Intensive Care Med 1996;22(10):1052–6.

[41] Wood G, MacLeod B, Moffatt S. Weaning from mechanical ventilation: physician-directed vs a respiratory-therapist-directed protocol. Respir Care 1995;40(3):219–24.

[42] Brower RG, Bernard G, Morris A. Ethics and standard of care in clinical trials. Am J Respir Crit Care Med 2004;170(2):198–9 [author reply 199].

[43] Weinert CR, Gross CR, Marinelli WA. Impact of randomized trial results on acute lung injury ventilator therapy in teaching hospitals. Am J Respir Crit Care Med 2003;167(10):1304–9.

[44] Young MP, Manning HL, Wilson DL, et al. Ventilation of patients with acute lung injury and acute respiratory distress syndrome: has new evidence changed clinical practice? Crit Care Med 2004; 32(6):1260–5.

[45] Randolph AG, Wypij D, Venkataraman ST, et al. Effect of mechanical ventilator weaning protocols on respiratory outcomes in infants and children: a randomized controlled trial. JAMA 2002;288(20): 2561–8.

[46] Ely EW, Bennett PA, Bowton DL, et al. Large scale implementation of a respiratory therapist-driven protocol for ventilator weaning. Am J Respir Crit Care Med 1999;159(2):439–46.

[47] Ventilation with lower tidal volumes as compared with traditional tidal volumes for acute lung injury and the acute respiratory distress syndrome. The Acute Respiratory Distress Syndrome Network. N Engl J Med 2000;342(18):1301–8.

[48] Brower RG, Lanken PN, MacIntyre N, et al. Higher versus lower positive end-expiratory pressures in patients with the acute respiratory distress syndrome. N Engl J Med 2004;351(4):327–36.

[49] Wiedemann HP, Wheeler AP, Bernard GR, et al. Comparison of two fluid-management strategies in acute lung injury. N Engl J Med 2006;354(24): 2564–75.

[50] Cabana MD, Rand CS, Powe NR, et al. Why don't physicians follow clinical practice guidelines? A framework for improvement. JAMA 1999;282(15): 1458–65.

[51] Burns SM, Marshall M, Burns JE, et al. Design, testing, and results of an outcomes-managed approach to patients requiring prolonged mechanical ventilation. Am J Crit Care 1998;7(1):45–57 [quiz: 58–9].

[52] Kollef MH, Shapiro SD, Clinkscale D, et al. The effect of respiratory therapist-initiated treatment protocols on patient outcomes and resource utilization. Chest 2000;117(2):467–75.

[53] Kollef MH, Shapiro SD, Silver P, et al. A randomized, controlled trial of protocol-directed versus

physician-directed weaning from mechanical ventilation. Crit Care Med 1997;25(4):567–74.

[54] Shrake KL, Scaggs JE, England KR, et al. Benefits
associated with a respiratory care assessment-
treatment program: results of a pilot study. Respir
Care 1994;39(7):715–24.

[55] Stoller JK, Haney D, Burkhart J, et al. Physician-
ordered respiratory care vs physician-ordered use
of a respiratory therapy consult service: early experience at The Cleveland Clinic Foundation. Respir
Care 1993;38(11):1143–54.

[56] Stoller JK, Mascha EJ, Kester L, et al. Randomized
controlled trial of physician-directed versus respiratory therapy consult service-directed respiratory
care to adult non-ICU inpatients. Am J Respir Crit
Care Med 1998;158(4):1068–75.

[57] Stoller JK, Skibinski CI, Giles DK, et al. Physician-
ordered respiratory care vs physician-ordered use of
a respiratory therapy consult service. Results of a prospective observational study. Chest 1996;110(2):
422–9.

[58] Krishnan JA, Moore D, Robeson C, et al. A
prospective, controlled trial of a protocol-based

strategy to discontinue mechanical ventilation. Am
J Respir Crit Care Med 2004;169(6):673–8.

[59] Marelich GP, Murin S, Battistella F, et al. Protocol
weaning of mechanical ventilation in medical and
surgical patients by respiratory care practitioners
and nurses: effect on weaning time and incidence of
ventilator-associated pneumonia. Chest 2000;
118(2):459–67.

[60] Scheinhorn DJ, Chao DC, Stearn-Hassenpflug M,
et al. Outcomes in post-ICU mechanical ventilation:
a therapist-implemented weaning protocol. Chest
2001;119(1):236–42.

[61] Cox CE, Carson SS, Ely EW, et al. Effectiveness of
medical resident education in mechanical ventilation. Am J Respir Crit Care Med 2003;167(1):32–8.

[62] Brochard L, Mancebo J, Wysocki M, et al. Noninvasive ventilation for acute exacerbations of chronic
obstructive pulmonary disease. N Engl J Med
1995;333(13):817–22.

[63] Kalhan R, Mikkelsen M, Dedhiya P, et al. Underuse
of lung protective ventilation: analysis of potential
factors to explain physician behavior. Crit Care
Med 2006;34(2):300–6.

ELSEVIER
SAUNDERS

Clin Chest Med 29 (2008) 323–328

CLINICS
IN CHEST
MEDICINE

Mechanical Ventilation in an Airborne Epidemic

Ghee-Chee Phua, MBBS, MRCP, FCCP[a,*], Joseph Govert, MD[b]

[a]Department of Respiratory and Critical Care Medicine, Singapore General Hospital,
Outram Road, Singapore 169608
[b]Division of Pulmonary, Allergy and Critical Care Medicine, Duke University,
Duke University Medical Center 31012, Durham, NC 27710, USA

The severe acute respiratory syndrome (SARS) outbreak of 2003 infected more than 8,000 people in 30 countries and killed more than 700 [1]. About 20% to 30% of SARS patients required admission to an intensive care unit (ICU), and most of them required mechanical ventilation [2]. SARS showed how swiftly infectious diseases can wreak havoc across the globe in the era of air travel. Most alarmingly, the initial pandemonium the SARS epidemic caused exposed how unprepared the medical community was for an airborne epidemic of this nature.

Currently, the threat of pandemic influenza is increasing, with the emergence of a highly virulent avian influenza virus, influenza A/H5N1 (AI H5N1). As of December 14, 2007, the World Health Organization (WHO) had reported 340 human cases of AI H5N1 in 13 countries, of which 208 (61%) have died [3]. There is concern that the acquisition of greater transmissibility by the virus may result in a replay of the Spanish flu, which killed 20 to 50 million people in 1918 [4]. In addition to the menace posed by emerging infectious diseases, a deliberate epidemic caused by a catastrophic bioterrorist attack remains a real and present danger [5].

SARS was an important wake-up call for the medical community and highlighted the need for increased preparedness to meet the looming threats of large-scale airborne epidemics. In these scenarios, intensive care providers will play a crucial role, as it is anticipated that a high proportion of victims will progress rapidly to respiratory failure and require mechanical ventilatory support.

This article explores many issues relating to mechanical ventilation in an airborne epidemic. The authors examine the lessons from SARS and consider the strategies for mechanical ventilation in future airborne epidemics, with special consideration given to the crucial issue of protection of the health care worker. Unfortunately, there is a paucity of evidence-based literature on the subject of mechanical ventilation in this setting, and it must be emphasized that most of the recommendations made are based largely on expert opinion pieces and retrospective reviews of the SARS experience.

Lessons from SARS

The SARS outbreak of 2003 was caused by a novel coronavirus [6]. It is believed that SARS originated in the exotic wildlife markets in southern China, where it crossed the species barrier from animal to man [7]. It first surfaced surreptitiously as an unusual cluster of 305 cases of atypical pneumonia, with at least five deaths in Guangdong province in November of 2002 [8]. Interestingly, this was initially thought to be because of chlamydia, and did not capture much attention.

The global SARS outbreak started on February 21, 2003, when a 65-year-old physician from Guangdong province arrived in Hong Kong to attend his daughter's wedding. He inadvertently infected at least 12 guests from six different countries at the hotel where he stayed. In the ensuing few months, SARS spread rapidly across 30 countries and infected more than 8,000 patients.

---

* Corresponding author.
E-mail address: phua.ghee.chee@sgh.com.sg
(G-C. Phua).

The worst hit regions were China, Hong Kong, Taiwan, Toronto (Canada), and Singapore. The morbidity, mortality, speed, and ease of transmission of SARS caught the medical community by surprise and exposed the lack of preparedness for dealing with an epidemic of this nature.

Approximately 20% to 30% of SARS patients required intensive care and mechanical ventilation for acute lung injury (ALI) and acute respiratory distress syndrome (ARDS) [9]. Among the critically ill SARS patients, approximately 50% died [10,11]. This placed a heavy burden on the staff and facilities of the ICU.

One of the alarming features of the SARS outbreak was nosocomial spread to health care workers caring for the critically ill. Around the world, at least 1,706 health care workers were stricken with SARS and a number died in the line of duty. In Singapore and Toronto, health care workers accounted for half of all SARS cases, and about 20% of critically ill SARS cases [12]. Tragically, one of the victims was Dr. Carlo Urbani of the WHO. Dr. Urbani was the physician who first alerted the world to SARS after being called to assist in the Hanoi outbreak [13]. He died of SARS on March 29, 2003. His foresight in swiftly recognizing the threat of SARS, and in issuing the global warning, saved many lives in Vietnam and around the world.

SARS taught the medical community several important lessons. It showed us how rapidly emerging infectious diseases in distant parts of the globe can reach our doorsteps in days, and highlighted the importance of global cooperation to contain infectious diseases. It demonstrated the vulnerability of health care facilities in an airborne epidemic, and the necessity of establishing stringent infection control measures and crisis management protocols. The high proportion of patients requiring mechanical ventilation alerted us to the ease at which an outbreak could overwhelm our critical care resources if we do not develop adequate surge capacity. Finally, SARS renewed our faith in the dedication of the medical professionals who care for patients, even at the risk of their own lives, while underlining the critical duty of health care administrators and senior physicians in instituting procedures to maximize the safety of frontline staff.

Strategies for mechanical ventilation

Approximately 20% of patients with SARS and most hospitalized patients with AI H5N1 progress rapidly to ALI or ARDS and require ventilatory support [14]. In an airborne epidemic caused by emerging infections or a bioterrorism event, it is envisaged that there will be a high incidence of hypoxemic respiratory failure because of ALI or ARDS, necessitating mechanical ventilation.

Lung protective ventilatory strategy

A low tidal volume lung protective strategy has been shown to improve survival in patients with ALI or ARDS [15]. Because most patients with ALI or ARDS do not die of refractory hypoxemia, this low tidal volume strategy likely improves outcome by reducing the systemic inflammatory response produced by ventilator-induced lung injury [16]. As the clinical and pathologic manifestations of SARS and AI H5N1 are indistinguishable from other causes of ALI or ARDS, and the cause of death is similarly refractory systemic inflammation, shock, and multiorgan failure, it seems reasonable that the ventilatory management principles learned in ALI and ARDS should be adopted in an airborne epidemic [9]. Thus, the authors recommend using volume or pressure control ventilation targeting tidal volumes of 6-mL/kg predicted body weight and plateau pressures of less than 30-cm of water. In addition, positive end expiratory pressure and fraction of inspired oxygen are adjusted to maintain a partial pressure of oxygen of 55 mm Hg to 80 mm Hg. Of particular note is the significant incidence of pneumothorax reported in patients with AI H5N1, which may necessitate a cautious approach to lung recruitment maneuvers [17].

Adjuvant strategies

Adjuvant strategies shown to decrease morbidity and mortality in critically ill patients on mechanical ventilation include deep venous thrombosis prophylaxis, stress ulcer prophylaxis, sedation protocols, and avoidance of neuromuscular blockage, if possible; semirecumbent position should also be employed during airborne epidemics causing hypoxemic respiratory failure [18]. While there were several reports on the use of corticosteroids in SARS and AI H5N1, there is insufficient evidence at this time to recommend their routine use [9,19].

High frequency oscillatory ventilation

There remains controversy regarding appropriate modes of ventilation for patients with refractory respiratory failure from highly infectious diseases. In particular, there are infection control concerns regarding aerosol generation with high-frequency oscillatory ventilation (HFOV) and the inability to filter exhaled air to the environment. There is currently little data available on the risk of disease transmission to health care workers from HFOV, and a retrospective study did not show a clear association between HFOV and SARS infection among health care workers, but the sample size was small and the verdict is still uncertain [20].

Noninvasive positive pressure ventilation

Similarly, there is debate about the use of noninvasive positive pressure ventilation (NIPPV). There have been reports of NIPPV being effective in treating patients with SARS and reducing the need for intubation [21]. This is an attractive option, especially in a pandemic scenario when the demand for mechanical ventilatory support is overwhelming. However, there are conflicting reports regarding its safety for health care workers [22]. There is worry about dispersion of infectious particles, and an experimental model confirmed substantial exposure to exhaled air occurring within 0.5 meters of patients receiving NIPPV [23]. Nevertheless, there were no reports of nosocomial transmission with adequate respiratory protection during SARS [19]. Patient selection is important for NIPPV, as it has not been shown to improve mortality in ARDS [24], and may not be suitable for patients where near-term improvement is not expected.

Protection of the health care worker

The heavy toll paid by health care workers during the SARS outbreak demonstrated the vulnerability of health care workers in a respiratory epidemic. The risk of transmission was particularly high in the ICU because of the high viral load in the critically ill, as well as aerosol-generating procedures, such as intubation, suctioning, and bronchoscopy. A retrospective cohort study reported a staggering 13-fold increase in the risk of becoming infected among health care workers who performed or assisted in endotracheal intubations [19].

The number of infected health care workers dropped dramatically after infection control measures were put in place, such as isolation of infected patients, use of personal protective equipment (PPE) for health care workers, and strict hand-hygiene for all [25]. WHO and the Centers

for Disease Control and Prevention (CDC) have issued guidelines that recommend the use of standard, contact, and airborne protection, including respirators of N95 standard or higher in an airborne epidemic [26,27]. Standard PPE includes N95 masks, gloves, gowns, caps, and face shields or goggles. All staff should be mask fit-tested to ensure an adequate seal. When performing high-risk procedures, such as intubation, bag-mask ventilation, or bronchoscopy, protection should be enhanced with powered air-purifying respirators.

In view of the high risk of disease transmission during endotracheal intubation, airway management protocols have been proposed [28]. Early intubation should be done, preferably in the ICU, rather than performing crash-intubation on the floor. Adequate sedation and neuromuscular blockade is recommended during intubation to minimize cough and dispersion of respiratory secretions. Finally, the procedure should be performed by the most experienced person available, both to minimize the dispersal of infectious particles and to reduce the number of individuals exposed during the intubation.

Other general recommendations include ensuring that the infectious disease ward is close to the ICU and that the ICU is equipped with negative pressure rooms. Aerosol-generating procedures should be avoided whenever possible. Measures to minimize respiratory droplet transmission include using in-line suctioning to maintain the ventilator circuit as a closed system. Humidification should be done via heat-moisture exchangers with viral-bacterial filter properties rather than heated humidifiers. Each ventilator should have two filters: one between the inspiratory port and ventilator circuit and the other between the expiratory port and ventilator circuit, to provide additional protection from exhaust gases and minimize ventilator contamination.

An essential component of infection-control strategy is staff training and the implementation of clear management protocols, including the use of PPE, monitoring staff health, quarantining staff, transport of patients, transfer to ICU, airway management, aerosol-generating procedures, environment and equipment disinfection, and visitation policies.

Pandemic scenario and preparations

For many years, public health officials have worried about a repeat of the Spanish influenza pandemic of 1918 to 1919, which infected

326 PHUA & GOVERT

approximately 500 million persons and killed 20 to 50 million [29]. In the United States, over a quarter of the population was infected, and some 675,000 died, or 10 times the number of Americans who died fighting in World War I [30].

There is little modern health care experience with respiratory mass casualties of this scale. However, it is apparent that the mortality, morbidity, and public confidence in the time of an airborne pandemic are likely to be highly dependent on the critical care response. It is therefore imperative for critical care providers to take the lead in planning and preparing for large-scale airborne epidemics and pandemics. Issues to be considered include developing triage protocols, augmenting ICU surge staffing, implementing rational infection control measures, stockpiling medical equipment and supplies, and information sharing among many units.

Surge capacity

Several recent publications have addressed the issue of expansion of intensive care in an epidemic [31–33]. Rubinson and colleagues [32] have recommended modifying usual standards of care, termed "emergency mass critical care practices," to maximize the number of patients treated. Others feel that over-stretching resources and deploying unfamiliar staff may backfire and result in staff infection, as well as a standard of care too poor to be of value. However, most investigators agree that there is a need to develop some surge capacity in response to an epidemic. Preparations include stockpiling positive pressure ventilators and medical supplies, adapting general hospital beds for critical care delivery, augmenting and training staff, enhancing infection control measures, and conducting preparedness exercises. To this end, many local, state, and national bodies have developed such stockpiles and disaster management plans. It is incumbent that all critical care practitioners be aware of these resources and plans . The Appendix lists resources for pandemic influenza planning and preparedness.

Triage

Despite our best preparations, it remains likely that in a pandemic scenario, the number of critically ill patients will overwhelm our critical care capacity. There is a need to develop triage protocols to prioritize access to limited resources, including mechanical ventilation [34]. Triage criteria should be based on clinical indicators of

survivability, and resources allocated to those most likely to benefit. These are difficult decisions and cannot be left until times of crisis. Development of triage protocols should be done in advance, with careful consideration of ethical principles [35]. It is crucial to engage the community in this process so that public trust exists when it is most needed.

Summary

With the increasing threat of pandemic influenza and catastrophic bioterrorism, it is important for intensive care providers to be prepared to meet the challenge of large-scale airborne epidemics causing mass casualty respiratory failure. The SARS outbreak exposed the vulnerability of health care workers and highlighted the importance of establishing stringent infection control and crisis management protocols. Patients with ALI or ARDS who require mechanical ventilation should receive a lung protective, low tidal volume strategy. There remains controversy regarding the use of HFOV and NIPPV. Standard, contact and airborne precautions should be instituted in the ICU, with special care taken when aerosol-generating procedures are performed. During an airborne pandemic, the mortality, morbidity, and public confidence are likely to be highly dependent on the critical care response. It is imperative for critical care providers to take the lead in planning and preparing for this eventuality.

Appendix

Web resources for pandemic influenza planning and preparedness

Official United States Government Web site for pandemic influenza: www.pandemicflu.gov

WHO epidemic and pandemic alert and response: www.who.int/csr/disease/influenza/pandemic/en

CDC Influenza Pandemic Operation Plan: www.cdc.gov/flu/pandemic/cdcplan.htm

Strategic National Stockpile: www.bt.cdc.gov/stockpile

United States State Government pandemic influenza resources: www.cidrap.umn.edu/cidrap/files/68/usplans.pdf

Singapore Influenza Pandemic Readiness and Response Plan: www.crisis.gov.sg/FLU

United Kingdom Department of Health: www.dh.gov.uk/en/PandemicFlu/index.htm

References

[1] World Health Organization. Summary of probable SARS cases with onset of illness from November 1, 2002 to July 31, 2003. Available at: http://www. who.int/csr/sars/country/table2004_04_21/en/index. html. Accessed December 18, 2007.

[2] Peiris JSM, Phil D, Yuen KY, et al. The severe acute respiratory syndrome. N Engl J Med 2003;349: 2431–41.

[3] World Health Organization. Cumulative number of confirmed human cases of avian influenza A/(H5N1) reported to WHO. Available at: http://www.who. int/csr/disease/avian_influenza/country/cases_table_ 2007_12_14/en/index.html. Accessed December 18, 2007.

[4] Tumpey TM, Basler CF, Aguilar PV, et al. Characterization of the reconstructed 1918 Spanish influenza pandemic virus. Science 2005;310:77–80.

[5] Karwa M, Bronzert P, Kvetan V. Bioterrorism and critical care. Crit Care Clin 2003;19(2):279–313.

[6] Ksiazek TG, Erdman D, Goldsmith CS, et al. A novel coronavirus associated with severe acute respiratory syndrome. N Engl J Med 2003;348: 1953–66.

[7] Guan Y, Zheng BJ, He YQ, et al. Isolation and characterization of viruses related to the SARS coronavirus from animals in southern China. Science 2003;302:276–8.

[8] Zhao Z, Zhang F, Xu M, et al. Description and clinical treatment of an early outbreak of severe acute respiratory syndrome (SARS) in Guangzhou, PR China. J Med Microbiol 2003;52:715–20.

[9] Levy MM, Baylor MS, Bernard GR, et al. Clinical issues and research in respiratory failure from severe acute respiratory syndrome. Am J Respir Crit Care Med 2005;171:518–26.

[10] Fowler RA, Lapinsky SE, Hallet D, et al, for the Toronto SARS Critical Care Group. Critically ill patients with severe acute respiratory syndrome. JAMA 2003;290:367–73.

[11] Lew TW, Kwek TK, Tai D, et al. Acute respiratory distress syndrome in critically ill patients with severe acute respiratory distress syndrome. JAMA 2003; 290:374–80.

[12] Booth CM, Matukas LM, Tomlinson GA, et al. Clinical features and short-term outcomes of 144 patients with SARS in the greater Toronto area. JAMA 2003;289:2801–9.

[13] Reilley B, Van Herp M, Sermand D, et al. SARS and Carlo Urbani. N Engl J Med 2003;348:1951–2.

[14] Beigel JH, Farrar J, Han AM, et al. Avian influenza A (H5N1) infection in humans. N Engl J Med 2005; 353:1374–85.

[15] The Acute Respiratory Distress Syndrome Network. Ventilation with lower tidal volumes as compared with traditional tidal volumes for acute lung injury and the acute respiratory distress syndrome. N Engl J Med 2000;342:1301–8.

[16] Parsons PE, Eisner MD, Thompson BT, et al. Lower tidal volume ventilation and plasma cytokine markers of inflammation in patients with acute lung injury. Crit Care Med 2005;33(1):1–6.

[17] Gruber PC, Gomersall CD, Joynt GM. Avian Influenza (H5N1): implications for intensive care. Intensive Care Med 2006;32:823–9.

[18] Dellinger RP, Carlet JM, Masur H, et al. Surviving sepsis campaign for management of severe sepsis and septic shock. Crit Care Med 2004;32:858–73.

[19] Arabi Y, Gomersall CD, Ahmed QA, et al. The critically-ill avian influenza A (H5N1) patient. Crit Care Med 2007;35:1397–403.

[20] Fowler RA, Guest CB, Lapinsky SE, et al. Transmission of severe acute respiratory syndrome during intubation and mechanical ventilation. Am J Respir Crit Care Med 2004;169:1198–202.

[21] Cheung TM, Yam LY, So LK, et al. Effectiveness of noninvasive positive pressure ventilation in the treatment of acute respiratory failure in severe acute respiratory syndrome. Chest 2004;126:845–50.

[22] Xiao Z, Li Y, Chen RC, et al. A retrospective study of 78 patients with severe acute respiratory syndrome. Chin Med J (Engl) 2003;116:805–10.

[23] Hui DS, Hall SD, Chan MT, et al. Noninvasive positive-pressure ventilation: an experimental model to assess air and particle dispersion. Chest 2006;130:730–40.

[24] Delclaux C, L'Her E, Alberti C, et al. Treatment of acute hypoxemic nonhypercapnic respiratory insufficiency with continuous positive airway pressure delivered by a face mask: a randomized controlled trial. JAMA 2000;284:2352–60.

[25] Low DE, McGeer A. SARS: one year later. N Engl J Med 2003;349:2381–2.

[26] World Health Organization. Avian Influenza, including influenza A (H5N1), in humans: WHO interim infection control guidelines for health care facilities. Available at: http://www.who.int/csr/ disease/avian_influenza/guidelines/infectioncontrol1/ en/index.html. Accessed December 18, 2007.

[27] Centers for Disease Control and Prevention. Interim recommendations for infection control in health care facilities caring for patients with known or suspected avian influenza. Available at: http://www.cdc.gov/ flu/avian/professional/infect-control.htm. Accessed December 18, 2007.

[28] Caputo KM, Byrick R, Chapman MG, et al. Intubation of SARS patients: infection and perspectives of healthcare workers. Can J Anesth 2006;53(2):122–9.

[29] Taubenger JK, Morens DM. 1918 influenza: the mother of all pandemics. Emerg Infect Dis 2006;12:15–22.

[30] Billings M. The influenza pandemic of 1918. Available at: www.stanford.edu/group/virus/uda. Accessed December 18, 2007.

[31] Gommersall CD, Tai DY, Loo S, et al. Expanding ICU facilities in an epidemic: recommendations based on experience from the SARS epidemic in Hong Kong and Singapore. Intensive Care Med 2006;32:1004–13.

[32] Rubinson L, Nuzzo JB, Talmor DS, et al. Augmentation of hospital critical care capacity after bioterrorist attack or epidemics: recommendations of the Working Group on Emergency Mass Critical Care. Crit Care Med 2005;33:2393–403.

[33] Daugherty EL, Branson R, Rubinson L. Mass casualty respiratory failure. Curr Opin Crit Care 2007;13:51–6.

[34] Christian MD, Hawryluck L, Wax RS, et al. Development of a triage protocol for critical care during an influenza pandemic. CMAJ 2006; 175(11):1377–81.

[35] Thompson AK, Faith K, Gibson JL, et al. Pandemic influenza preparedness: an ethical framework to guide decision-making. BMC Medical Ethics 2006;7:12.

ELSEVIER
SAUNDERS

CLINICS
IN CHEST
MEDICINE

Clin Chest Med 29 (2008) 329–342

Proportional Assist Ventilation and Neurally Adjusted Ventilatory Assist—Better Approaches to Patient Ventilator Synchrony?

Christer Sinderby, PhD[a,b,*], Jennifer Beck, PhD[c,d]

[a]Department of Critical Care Medicine, Keenan Research Centre, Li Ka Shing Knowledge Institute,
St. Michael's Hospital, 30 Bond Street, Queen Wing 4-072, Toronto, Ontario, Canada M5B1W8
[b]Department of Medicine, University of Toronto, Toronto, Ontario, Canada
[c]Department of Newborn and Developmental Paediatrics, Neonatal Intensive Care Unit, Sunnybrook Health Sciences
Centre, Women's College Campus, 76 Grenville Street, Toronto, Ontario, Canada M5S 1B2
[d]Department of Pediatrics, University of Toronto, Toronto, Ontario, Canada

Breathing is a complex bodily function that allows oxygen to enter the body, carbon dioxide to leave the body, and regulates pH by maintaining adequate ventilation during rest, exercise, sleep, and other activities. Breathing is affected by speech, emotions, discomfort, and pain. To soothe the latter, sedation and analgesia are often used at the price of affecting the respiratory drive. Understanding the regulation of breathing in the critical care patient is thus multifaceted, especially in ventilator-dependent patients who must interact with artificial respiration.

Mechanical ventilation originally consisted of simple, manually-driven pump devices (mainly used for resuscitation), but has developed into advanced positive pressure ventilators for continuous support of patients in respiratory failure. This evolution has resulted in mechanical ventilators that deliver assist intermittently, attempting to mimic natural breathing. The crudest forms deliver fixed volumes or pressures with fixed rates and breath durations, while more advanced modes allow the patient to trigger the ventilator with their own effort, which can then be cycled-off on time criteria or when certain flow criteria have been met. Recently, modes of mechanical ventilation that synchronize not only the timing, but also the level of assist to the patient's own effort have been introduced, such as proportional assist ventilation (PAV) [1,2] and neurally adjusted ventilatory assist (NAVA) [3]. This article describes the concepts related to PAV and NAVA, and how they relate to conventional modes in terms of patient-ventilator synchrony.

International use reviews indicate that about one third of adult intensive care unit (ICU) patients receive mechanical ventilation for about 1 week [4,5]. A recent study involving 253 United States hospitals shows that mechanical ventilation increases daily costs by approximately $1,500 per day for patients receiving treatment in the ICU throughout their entire stay [6]. Sedatives are universally used in critically ill and mechanically-ventilated patients, and their use is associated with a longer duration of mechanical ventilation,

Dr. Sinderby and Dr. Beck have made inventions related to neural control of mechanical ventilation that are patented. The license for these patents belongs to Maquet Critical Care. Future commercial uses of this technology may provide financial benefit to Dr. Sinderby and Dr. Beck through royalties. Dr. Sinderby and Dr. Beck each own 50% of Neurovent Research Inc., a research and development company that builds the equipment and catheters for research studies. Neurovent Research Inc. has a consulting agreement with Maquet Critical Care.

* Corresponding author. Department of Critical Care Medicine, Keenan Research Centre, Li Ka Shing Knowledge Institute, St. Michael s Hospital, 30 Bond Street, Queen Wing 4-072, Toronto, Ontario, Canada M5B1W8.
E-mail address: sinderbyc@smh.toronto.on.ca (C. Sinderby).

weaning time, and length of stay in the ICU [7,8]. In addition, the choice of sedatives impacts on the duration of mechanical ventilation [9]. Although use of sedatives is to relieve stress and reduce discomfort in critically ill patients, daily sedative interruption does not result in adverse psychologic outcomes, and actually indicates a positive impact on posttraumatic stress disorder [10].

When considering the relevance of patient-ventilator interaction, Thille and colleagues recently demonstrated that patient-ventilator asynchrony is associated with a prolonged duration of mechanical ventilation [11,12]. Asynchrony also causes sleep disruption [13] in adult patients. In neonates, systematic reviews suggest shorter duration of ventilation as one benefit for patient-triggered ventilation [14]. It was mentioned that

because of lack of respiratory monitoring, it was not possible to conclude that the mechanism of producing those benefits is by the actual provocation of synchronized ventilation.

Transmission of respiratory motoneuron output to ventilation: the neuroventilatory coupling

To recognize the complexity of patient-ventilator interaction, the chain-of-events that take place during spontaneous breathing are presented in Fig. 1 and explained in the rest of this section.

Voluntary and involuntary control of the respiratory muscles originate from separate sites in the central nervous system and have separate descending pathways. Voluntary control arises from the motor and premotor cortex, whereas

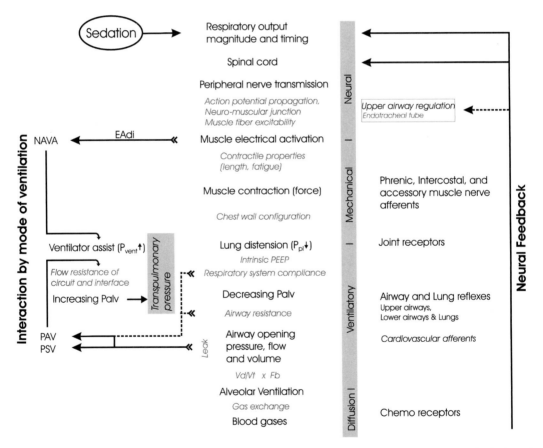

Fig. 1. Schematic description of the chain of events during spontaneous breathing and interaction to mechanical ventilation. The center panel describes the transformation steps from central initiation of a breath to the generation of airway pressure, flow, and volume. The right panel indicates the neural feedback systems involved in the control of breathing. The left panel shows at which level and how different modes of mechanical ventilation interact during spontaneous breathing. EAdi, electrical activity of the diaphragm; Fb, breathing frequency; Palv, alveolar pressure; P_{pl}, pleural pressure; PSV, pressure support ventilation; P_{vent}, ventilator pressure; V_D, dead space; V_T, tidal volume.

involuntary control is mediated by both rhythmic and nonrhythmic systems located in the brainstem.

These control systems integrate at segmental levels in the spinal cord, where descending information from these systems is modulated by reflexes [15]. The respiratory motoneuron output is then transmitted to respiratory muscles via motor nerves and neuromuscular junctions [16], which initiates action potential propagation along the muscle fibers. In the case of the diaphragm, the principle inspiratory muscle, this action potential propagation along the muscle fibers is the source of the electrical activity of the diaphragm (EAdi), a signal whose strength will depend on the number of motor units recruited and their firing rate [17]. To put the rapidity of this signal transmission into perspective, the latency time from stimulation of the phrenic nerve in the neck to the onset of the diaphragm compound muscle action potential in healthy subjects is about 6 ms to 8 ms, [16,18,19].

The EAdi starts the contractile machinery of the muscle cells and shortening of the muscle. The inspiratory muscles will act to expand the thorax by generating negative pressure around the lungs, which in turn act to distend the lung parenchyma and lower the alveolar pressure. If the airways are patent, inspiratory flow will commence when airway and alveolar pressures are lower than the pressure at the airway opening. In healthy subjects, the time for the transmission of neural output to onset of mechanical output is in the 20-ms range [20].

In disease, the time required to transform neural output into airway flow can be drastically prolonged. Neural disorders can impair nerve conduction [16,18], reduce the number of conducting nerves, and impair neuromuscular transmission. Muscular disorders or hostile intra- or extracellular cellular milieus can delay excitation of and reduce the number of muscle cells being excited. In addition, they can impair the contractile machinery within the muscle cell and reduce force generation. Shorter muscle length and altered chest-wall configuration (eg, because of hyperinflation) impair the muscle force, as well as its transformation into the negative pleural pressure that is necessary to expand the lungs [17]. Dynamic hyperinflation imposes a threshold load, also called intrinsic positive end-expiratory pressure (PEEP), and may induce substantial delays between onset of effort and inspiratory flow [21].

A reduced lung compliance and presence of airway obstruction adds extra load to inflate the lungs, requiring extra efforts in spontaneously breathing patients. The resulting alveolar ventilation then depends on the tidal volume, dead space, and breathing frequency. Depending on the alveolar-capillary interface, gases will be exchanged with the blood. Hence, a deficiency at any of the above steps converting neural motor output into ventilation can delay, reduce, or block the signals used to control the ventilator and thus induce acute respiratory failure.

Neural feedback from the respiratory system

Respiration is regulated by a very complete feedback system, including many reflex loops, which are often not considered in the clinical application of mechanical ventilation of spontaneously breathing patients.

Lungs

The lungs host stretch-sensitive receptors and respond to lung distension, which is dominantly mediated by vagal afferents. Based on the response to sustained lung distension, these receptors are divided into rapidly adapting (RAR) and slowly adapting (SAR) receptors. SARs are sensitive to lung inflation and adjust the breathing pattern by shortening inspiration and prolonging expiration (Hering-Breuer reflex) [22]. RARs are stimulated by lung inflation and deflation and are activated by mechanical stimulus, such as changes in lung compliance, as well as by chemical stimuli. The described reflex responses of RARs are augmented breaths, tachypnea, and cough. Bronchial C-fiber receptors are affected by tissue damage, pulmonary edema, inflammatory and immunologic mediators, and inhaled irritants. Described respiratory responses for bronchial C-fiber receptors include apnea or rapid shallow breathing and cough. Neuroepithelial bodies are cells thought to be activated during hypoxia and exert local actions on airway smooth muscles and bronchial and pulmonary vascular beds, for example. The role of their function has yet to be clarified. For complete reviews, the reader is referred to the works of Widdicombe [23,24] and Undem and Kollarik [25].

Upper airways

There are several sensory receptors in the larynx, including pressure receptors, cold receptors, irritant receptors, and C-fiber receptors [23,24]. There is also evidence that recruitment of laryngeal, tongue, and hyoid muscles during airway obstruction is influenced by slowly adapting pulmonary stretch receptors [26]. The role of these receptors during mechanical ventilation will of course depend on whether or not an endo-tracheal tube is present.

Muscle afferents

It has long been understood that the respiratory muscles have significant proprioceptive innervation, although there are clear differences between the respiratory muscles [27–29]. Animal studies have revealed a number of phrenic afferent responses to electrical or chemical stimulus, such as changes in phrenic nerve efferent drive and altered breathing pattern and ventilation, also known as phrenic-to-phrenic reflex [30–33], or changes in the drive to intercostal muscles, also known as intercostal-to-phrenic reflex [34,35]. Reflex responses mediated by receptors, which most likely lie within the costovertebral joints, have also been suggested as the primary determinant of the load-compensating reflex [36]. Although information mainly pertains to animal data, it is thought that phrenic afferents have little influence on respiratory muscle activity during eupneic breathing; however, when activated by mechanical or chemical stimuli, they can reflexively alter efferent drive to the diaphragm [37].

Chemoreceptors

Chemoreceptors are ultimately responsible for maintenance of constant levels of arterial P_{O2}, P_{CO2} and [H$^+$], protecting the brain from hypoxia and ensuring that the breathing is always appropriate for metabolism. The peripheral chemoreceptors in the carotid bodies respond primarily to hypoxemia, whereas central chemoreceptors in the brainstem respond to hypercapnia. Activation of either the hypoxic or hypercapnic chemoreflex elicits both hyperventilation and sympathetic activation. (For review, see Refs. [38,39]).

Integration of a mechanical ventilator

Mechanical ventilation mainly accomplishes two tasks: it provides adequate ventilation and it unloads the respiratory muscles. If mechanical ventilation is applied without coordination to inspiratory muscle activity (asynchronous), ventilation can reduce respiratory drive primarily via a chemoreceptor response. If the assist is delivered

synchronously with inspiratory effort, it will overcome increased elastic and resistive loads and compensate for muscle weakness.

To ensure that assist is delivered in synchrony with patient effort, appropriate monitoring is required. Waveform analysis of flow, pressure, and volume tracings have been suggested (for a complete review, see Ref. [40]); however, these methods are limited. For example, the PSV tracing on the left side in Fig. 2 actually indicates wasted inspiratory efforts in a patient not using his diaphragm at all. New indices to detect poor triggering and timing of assist have recently been published [41,42]. Even though timing is important, information about respiratory drive is perhaps more important because asynchrony can lead to increased efforts [43] by loading the diaphragm and the other inspiratory muscles during delayed triggering or wasted efforts. The introduction of esophageal pressure measurements on some mechanical ventilators can provide information about lung distending pressures and unloading. Monitoring of EAdi can provide information about synchrony in terms of timing and magnitude of the assist, as well as make it possible to observe if respiratory drive is reduced with increased assist.

To discuss how mechanical ventilators interact with spontaneously breathing patients, four features can be described: triggering of assist, delivery of assist, cycling-off assist, and expiration.

Triggering of assist

Impaired triggering of the ventilator increases the amount of work to start the ventilator [44,45] and can be associated with discomfort and changes in the cerebral cortex activation [46]. Conventional ventilators are predominantly equipped with pneumatic trigger systems sensitive to changes in airway pressure, flow, or volume. Consequently, with a pneumatic trigger, assist can only be initiated after all transformations outlined for the neuroventilatory coupling have taken place (see Fig. 1). If the impairment of the neuroventilatory coupling is proximal to the level where changes in airway pressure, flow, or volume occur, a winning strategy to obtain best triggering is to measure the trigger signal as close to the respiratory centers as possible and eliminate the steps where the trigger delays occur.

The most proximal level where a neural trigger signal can be obtained is currently at the level of the electrical activation of the diaphragm (see

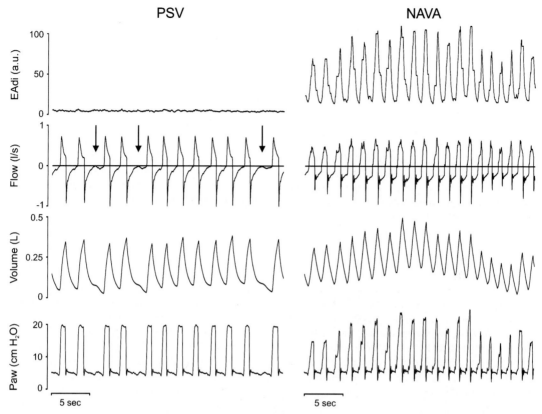

Fig. 2. Comparison of PSV and NAVA in a patient who has respiratory failure. From top to bottom: Diaphragm electrical activity, flow, volume, and airway pressure (Paw) in a patient who has respiratory failure on PSV (*left panel*) and NAVA (*right panel*). All delivered breaths were triggered during PSV period and as indicated by the arrows, there were also indications of wasted inspiratory efforts in the flow and pressure tracings. The EAdi, however, indicated that the diaphragm was not active at all during PSV (*left panel*). After switching the patient to NAVA, diaphragm activity was restored (*right panel*), suggesting that the patient ventilator asynchrony was caused by overassist during PSV and that waveform analysis of flow and pressure without EAdi may be misleading. (*Reprinted from* Sinderby C, Brander L, Beck J. Is one fixed level of assist sufficient to mechanically ventilate spontaneously breathing patients? In: Vincent JL, editor. Yearbook of intensive care and emergency medicine. Berlin: Springer Verlag; 2007. p. 348–57; with permission.)

Fig. 1) [3,47]. The EAdi can be measured with microelectrodes placed on a nasogastric tube in the esophagus [3]. Although, disorders affecting nerves, neuromuscular junction, and muscle excitability weaken the EAdi signal, they also weaken the pneumatic signaling. Studies in severe neuromuscular diseases still suggest that the EAdi signal is better protected from delays and dampening relative to pneumatic signals [48,49].

If the neuroventilatory coupling is optimal, the time delay from the onset of neural output to the generation of airway pressure, flow, and volume is very short and differences in trigger response time between PSV, PAV, and NAVA should be clinically indifferent, unless trigger sensitivities are set inadequately. It has been studied whether pressure or flow triggering is better [45,50] and results seem to favor flow triggering; however, whether this discussion is more of an academic issue than a clinical one is debatable.

The EAdi signal used with NAVA represents well the global diaphragm activity in both healthy subjects [17] and mechanically ventilated patients with acute respiratory failure [47]. A unique feature of pneumatic trigger systems is that they respond to global muscle efforts, to which the contribution of different muscle groups may vary. To match this, an ideal neural trigger would have to sense neural activation of all inspiratory muscles. Although the diaphragm is regarded as the principal inspiratory muscle, and the EAdi signal used with NAVA represents its activation [17,47], situations of increased respiratory demand in patients with acute respiratory failure also call for extra-diaphragmatic muscle recruitment, to offset the effects of increased load [51,52]. The combined implementation of neural and pneumatic trigger during NAVA overcomes this problem of non-diaphragmatic pretrigger efforts.

The most powerful factor impairing the neuroventilatory coupling (see Fig. 1) and hampering pneumatic triggering of mechanical ventilation is intrinsic PEEP [12,53,54]. Intrinsic PEEP is associated with dynamic hyperinflation, shortening of the inspiratory muscles, and an unfavorable chest wall configuration, reducing the diaphragm pressure generating efficiency [55], as well as imposing an inspiratory threshold load dampening and delaying the pneumatic trigger signal. Because the EAdi takes place before the mechanical induction of intrinsic PEEP (see Fig. 1), the EAdi signal is not delayed or dampened [55]. With regards to PAV, the patient-controlled assist delivery should theoretically suggest a reduced potential for dynamic hyperinflation and intrinsic PEEP. However, studies in chronic obstructive pulmonary disease (COPD) indicate a strong dependency of applied PEEP to compensate for intrinsic PEEP [56].

The most delicate problem during mechanical ventilation is probably to maintain a good comfort level, where the patient is adequately unloaded but still performing breathing efforts. Sedation and hyperventilation are powerful factors influencing the respiratory drive, especially when combined. Reduced respiratory drive (because of sedation) decreases trigger efforts, which promotes ineffective trigger attempts, and if compensated by a more sensitive trigger setting may induce autotriggering, where the ventilator's trigger may sense nonbreathing-related signals (eg, because of a cardiogenic induced mechanical oscillation) [57]. With time cycled modes, autotriggering could increase the ventilator rate and cause hyperventilation. During PSV, autotriggering would deliver breaths, and the volume delivered would depend on the level of PSV, the sensitivity setting of the flow off-cycling algorithm (see below). If settings are inappropriate (eg, trigger too sensitive, assist is too high and, off-cycling too insensitive), PSV can turn into a quasi-pressure control device and hyperventilate the patient to apnea (see Fig. 2).

Similar to PSV, PAV may experience autotriggering; however, because of the flow and volume-dependent control of assist delivery, small artifacts

(eg, from cardiac contractions) should only result in brief periods of low assist if PAV levels are set adequately. If the EAdi trigger used with NAVA is set too sensitively, NAVA can also be triggered by nonbreathing-related signals, such as an ECG (electrical) signal leaking into the EAdi signal. However, different from PSV, NAVA would cycle-off immediately after the alien signal had ceased, such that this trigger would occur during every ECG leak-through, causing brief period of assist. If ECG-false triggering during NAVA is excessive, the breathing frequency would match the heart rate (which is detected by algorithms and causes an alarm).

Another frequent problem with triggering is the presence of leaks in the respiratory circuit or between the patient and the ventilator circuit interface, which will call for increased flow delivery to maintain expiratory pressure in the respiratory circuit and, if too excessive, cause a decrease in the circuit pressure. Consequently if set too sensitively, a flow trigger is affected by leaks. In the presence of larger leaks, pressure and volume-sensitive triggers may be affected, depending on their settings [58]. As depicted in Fig. 1, leaks affect flow and volume and occur later in the neuroventilatory coupling than the onset of Eadi; hence, neural triggering is not influenced by leaks [59].

In clear contrast to triggered ventilation is controlled mechanical ventilation, where the respiratory rate and breath duration is fixed. Instead of obtaining the ultimate asynchrony, as perhaps would be expected, studies have shown that implementing a ventilator rate different from that of the patient often results in the patient adapting to the rate of the ventilator, also known as entrainment [60]. The underlying physiologic mechanisms of entrainment are becoming better understood and may suggest a clinical value where the patient is synchronized to the ventilator and not the other way around, as is the case with synchronized modes of mechanical ventilation [61]. However, in the event that entrainment is unsuccessful [62], there is still a demand for systems to monitor the ventilator-patient interaction.

Cycling-off the assist

Pneumatic off-cycling algorithms are designed to sense a decrease in flow relative to the peak inspiratory flow. This makes the off-cycling affected by the ratio of time constant of the respiratory system to patient neural inspiratory time, and the ratio of the pressure support to maximal inspiratory muscle pressure [63]. Note that recruitment of expiratory muscles is not taken into consideration.

According to the equation of Yamada and Du [63], when the patient inspiratory pressure generation is predominant (as compared with the ventilator support pressure), the ventilator is predisposed to be in synchrony with the patient's expiration. In contrast, when ventilator support overwhelms the patient inspiratory effort, expiratory asynchrony may easily occur. Depending on the patient mechanics, fixed levels of the flow termination criterion can cause the off-cycling to be synchronized or asynchronized (premature or delayed) with respect to the neural breath termination. In general terms, increasing PSV levels results in delayed off-cycling [43,64] and wasted inspiratory efforts [43,65]. These factors vary between diseases and vary on a breath-by-breath basis. Consequently, the flow termination criteria required to obtain synchronized off-cycling during PSV has been found to be very different between different patient categories [66,67]. To increase complexity, a recent study also showed that appropriately adjusted off-cycling criteria during PSV had a beneficial effect on reducing intrinsic PEEP in COPD: that is, it would improve the triggering [68]. Delayed off-cycling has also been shown to interfere with the natural breathing pattern of intubated adults [69] and infants [70].

Leaks in the patient-ventilator interface would hamper the decrease of flow and delay the flow-based off-cycling used with PSV. If leaks are excessive, this would cause inability to cycle-off assist, a so called "hang-up" [58].

Similar to PSV, PAV is also cycled-off by flow; however, different from PSV, assist is proportional to effort, keeping the ratio between assist and effort constant. If compensation for elastance and resistance is adequate, PAV will cease increasing assist when inspiratory effort stops, promoting a more synchronized off-cycling [71]. If compensation for elastance and resistance is too high, PAV may delay off-cycling and cause so called "run-away" [65].

Similar to PSV, PAV is affected by leaks in the patient-ventilator interface and may result in impaired off-cycling. From a theoretic perspective, unavoidable control-system delay during PAV has been suggested to influence expiratory asynchrony during PAV [72].

During NAVA, off-cycling algorithms are designed to sense a decrease in EAdi relative to the peak EAdi, a process which takes place early in the neuroventilatory coupling and hence, is not flow dependent (see Fig. 1). It should be noted that respiratory system mechanics still plays a role in the timing of neural off-cycling and reversal of flow [63]. Therefore, NAVA also has the ability to pneumatically cycle-off the assist if the pressure sensed by the ventilator exceeds the targeted pressure. In an animal model of acute lung injury, neural cycling-off has recently been shown to be unaffected by leaks [59].

Assist delivery

During spontaneous breathing, flow and volume, as well as inspiratory efforts, vary between breaths because of emotional, conscious influences or metabolic demand, or load. This takes place during ventilatory assist as well, except with the difference that the assist delivery will affect the breathing pattern in a variety of ways as well [64,70,73–77], and that responses to load or assist can vary whether perceived or not [78].

PSV does not respond to changes in inspiratory effort, and therefore the assist level, inspiratory rise time, and off-cycling criteria must be set manually and frequently to optimize assist [79]. Although this allows manipulation of the breathing pattern in many ways, which may be of advantage, it may also result in over- or under assist of the patient from time to time, as the respiratory demand, inspiratory load, muscle function, dynamic hyperinflation, and other factors change. Complex control loops have recently been introduced to automatically regulate the level of assist with conventional modes.

Volume-targeted modes introduce algorithms designed to maintain a constant tidal volume at the lowest pressure and are applied in spontaneously breathing patients to control tidal volume during PSV, for example, especially in neonatal and pediatric care [80,81]. The left panel of Fig. 3 illustrates an example of volume-targeted pressure support, where increasing spontaneous breathing efforts are associated with decreasing assist in a premature baby on pressure support with volume-targeted ventilation. The right panel shows how the assist responds to increasing inspiratory effort during NAVA. From patient ventilator interaction, perspective volume-targeted modes may actually deliver assist in inverse proportion to the patient's inspiratory effort. The influence of volume-targeted modes of mechanical ventilation on unloading of the respiratory muscles and

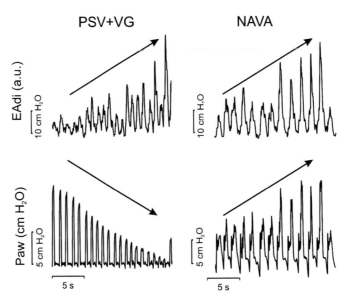

Fig. 3. Principle differences in patient-ventilator interaction between volume-targeted ventilation and proportional-assisted modes. Volume-targeted ventilation mode is shown on the left panel and proportional assisted mode is shown on the right panel. The figure demonstrates tracings of EAdi (*top*) and airway pressure (*bottom*) in an intubated premature infant. Note that during PSV plus volume guarantee (VG), as the diaphragm activity increases, the airway pressure is actually decreasing (reversed proportionality). During NAVA, the airway pressure increases in proportion to the EAdi.

impact on the breathing pattern has not yet been described. In addition, there are no randomized controlled trials showing the value of volume-targeted strategies in neonatology [82]. Furthermore, the reliability of algorithms used to control the volume-targeted assist has been discussed [80].

Adaptive support ventilation (ASV) is an automatic ventilation mode in which minute volume is controlled by a combination of tidal volume and breathing frequency, based on respiratory mechanics according to the Otis and colleagues equation [83]. In patients unable to trigger a breath, the ventilator generates pressure-controlled breaths and adjusts the inspiratory pressure and the timing to achieve the target tidal volume and breathing frequency. In spontaneously breathing patients, PSV will automatically be adjusted to achieve the target tidal volume [83]. Recent work has shown that ASV selects different tidal volume-breathing frequency combinations based on respiratory mechanics in a patient who does not trigger the ventilator. However, this was not the case when patients triggered the ventilator [84].

Traditionally, adjustment of mechanical ventilation aims to reduce rapid shallow breathing (often associated with acute respiratory failure), which means to reduce breathing frequency, increase tidal volume, and improve ventilation and

P_{CO2} to "comfort" levels. Dojat and colleagues [85] introduced a closed-loop knowledge-based system for driving PSV to achieve a respiratory pattern of comfort. The system automatically maintains the pressure support level at a minimum, while ensuring that tidal volume remains above a minimum threshold, end-tidal carbon dioxide level below a maximum threshold, and respiratory rate within a given range [85,86]. A randomized controlled trial compared this computer-driven system to a physician-controlled weaning process and demonstrated a reduction in mechanical ventilation duration and ICU length of stay by approximately 40% [86].

There are no reports on patient-ventilator synchrony during closed-loop control of PSV. However, it is known that changes in PSV modulate the breathing pattern in a predictive manner, where increasing PSV typically increases the tidal volume and decreases respiratory rate. The underlying cause is delayed off-cycling (assist that persists into neural exhalation), which prolongs neural exhalation and hence, reduces the respiratory rate [64,69,70]. The underlying mechanism for the outcome of closed loop systems for PSV adjustment [84,86] may therefore be uniquely related to the off-cycling algorithm of PSV.

Moreover, increases in the level of PSV are associated with increases in the rate of ineffective triggering [44,65,87], which if excessive, may increase the inspiratory muscle effort despite increasing PSV levels [43]. Conversely, reduction of the PSV level to eliminate ineffective triggering is frequently poorly tolerated by patients [12]. In other words, during PSV complex interference between trigger, cycling-off, and assist delivery may impose a limit to its use [87].

Different from PSV, neither NAVA [43,88–90] nor PAV [1,91–93] alter tidal volume or respiratory rate to the same extent when assist levels are modified. Instead, effort controlled modes show that within each patient, in a given state, there exist unique values for a desired minute ventilation, tidal volume, and breathing frequency that are largely independent of the mechanical load; if assist is increased, patient effort is decreased if not in demand.

PAV is a mode allowing the ventilator to amplify the patient instantaneous effort throughout inspiration while the patient controls the breathing pattern. This approach is implemented by monitoring the instantaneous rate and volume of gas flow from ventilator to patient. The applied pressure changes according to the equation of motion, using appropriately selected functions for the relation between pressure and volume and pressure and flow [1]. Fig. 1 indicates where PAV is located on the neuroventilatory coupling sequence; the solid and dashed lines indicate continuously and intermittently measured values, respectively.

PAV has been demonstrated to unload respiratory muscles [93] to the same level as PSV [56,94,95], and compensates for added respiratory load and hypercapnic stimulus better than PSV [96–98], with similar clinically comparable short-term effects on gas exchange and hemodynamics [99,100]. At too high levels of assist, PAV develops runaway phenomena (see off-cycling) [65].

In neonates, PAV safely maintains gas exchange at lower mean airway pressures and lower transpulmonary pressure changes, compared with patient-triggered ventilation (A/C intermittent mandatory ventilation), without adverse effects in this population [101,102]. Extremely premature infants who are supported by PAV breathe with a tidal volume of approximately 5 mL/kg, maintain carbon dioxide levels, and modify their spontaneous breathing in response to changes in thermal environment, such that P_{CO2} levels are appropriately maintained early in postnatal life [103]. The incidence and duration of respiratory pauses were not different with PAV.

In addition, in the adult patient, PAV has been reported to require lower airway pressure for unloading than with PSV and intermittent positive pressure ventilation [104,105]. Mitrouska and colleagues [106] showed that during carbon dioxide stimulus, neuroventilatory coupling was better preserved with proportional-assist ventilation than with pressure-support and assist-volume control ventilation. More variable tidal volumes with PAV indicate an increased ability of the patients to respond to alterations in respiratory demand vis-à-vis PSV [94,107].

For accurate application of PAV, it is important to assess the compliance and resistance of the patient and the endotracheal tube, so that levels of unloading that fully compensate for the resistance and compliance levels can be avoided. This may be of particular interest in neonates [108]. Recent implementation of algorithms that frequently sense elastance [109] and resistance [110] have a propensity to overcome these limitations [111].

Because PAV is patient driven, significant central inhibition of the respiratory drive (eg, because of excessive sedation) may impede assist delivery and ventilation. During PAV, leaks providing erroneous readings of flow and volume would be deleterious; however, PAV has been reported to be successfully implemented noninvasively and appreciated as more comfortable than conventional modes [112–118].

In its current platform, NAVA uses the EAdi to control the assist delivery above PEEP. PAV, on the other hand, uses a surrogate measurement of respiratory output to control mechanical ventilation, which is located further down the line of the neuroventilatory coupling (see Fig. 1). To the authors' knowledge, there are no studies comparing the EAdi to predicted respiratory muscle pressure during PAV, using a reliable EAdi methodology. Such a study would provide valuable information regarding the similarities and differences between NAVA and PAV.

During NAVA, both the ventilator and the patient's diaphragm receive the same electrical activation. Therefore, NAVA is inherently different than other modes in that the ventilator follows the patient's neural output directly and throughout each inspiration [3,119]. If the respiratory centers sense and respond to changes in inspiratory load and inspiratory muscle weakness, this will regulate the pressure-assist level [119]. Thus, NAVA can be considered as a mode that empowers the patient's diaphragm function, acting as an artificial muscle. During PAV, acute changes in respiratory system mechanics need to be accounted for.

In addition to responding to changes in respiratory load, NAVA also responds to increasing lung volumes. During lung distension, stretch-sensitive receptors feedback to the respiratory centers and terminate neural inspiration, thereby cycling-off the assist [88]. Interestingly, in sedated patients with acute respiratory failure, the spontaneously chosen tidal volume is approximately 6 mL/kg (personal body weight) [89], a tidal volume considered to be lung protective [120].

With respect to unloading, different from both PSV and PAV, NAVA can be applied at levels of assist that eliminate the work of breathing without causing patient-ventilator asynchrony or the elimination of the EAdi (the controller signal) [88,119].

Because the ventilator is controlled by respiratory drive, during NAVA the use of sedatives, analgesics, and other central depressants or stimulants may have an impact on the EAdi. Given that NAVA allows monitoring of assist, ventilation, patient ventilator synchrony, and changes in neural respiratory drive, it is possible to evaluate if the patient is being suitably ventilated with NAVA or not. NAVA is the only mode that actually makes it possible to monitor and quantify the respiratory drive to the diaphragm through online display of EAdi.

Leaks during NAVA will not affect the accuracy of assist delivery unless the leak is so large that the targeted pressure cannot be obtained. However, the NAVA level may have to be increased to compensate for the efficiency of assist delivery during leaks [59].

Expiration

Little is known about the expiratory side of asynchrony. Beck and colleagues [47,70] showed in both infant and adult patients that ventilator assist frequently continues after the diaphragm activity has ceased (ie, into neural exhalation). Jubran and colleagues [121] demonstrated expiratory efforts in 5 of 12 subjects with COPD before the cessation of inspiratory flow, signifying that the subject was "fighting" the ventilator at breathing frequencies less than 30 breaths per minute. Parthasarathy and colleagues [122] showed that the continuation of mechanical inflation into neural expiration was associated with failure of the subsequent inspiratory attempt to trigger the ventilator. These data suggest that the expiratory period and recruitment of expiratory muscles also add to the complexity of patient-ventilator interaction.

Summary

Patient-ventilator interaction is a complex topic, where interaction between patient effort, triggering, assist levels, off-cycling, and sedation all play a role. Patient-ventilator asynchrony prolongs the duration of mechanical ventilation and this may be interrelated with sedation practice. It is therefore important to raise the awareness of how mechanical ventilation affects breathing pattern and effort via on-line monitoring, allowing us to better understand how to best tailor the assist with regards to synchrony, effort, and breathing pattern, and to appreciate the power of mechanical ventilation in spontaneously breathing patients. There is also need for monitors and alarms to detect patient-ventilator asynchrony in the clinic. Finally, there is no doubt that PAV and NAVA appear superior to conventional modes of mechanical ventilation in terms of delivering assist in synchrony with patient efforts.

References

[1] Younes M. Proportional assist ventilation, a new approach to ventilatory support. Theory. Am Rev Respir Dis 1992;145(1):114–20.

[2] Younes M, Puddy A, Roberts D, et al. Proportional assist ventilation. Results of an initial clinical trial. Am Rev Respir Dis 1992;145(1):121–9.

[3] Sinderby C, Navalesi P, Beck J, et al. Neural control of mechanical ventilation in respiratory failure. Nat Med 1999;5:1433–6.

[4] Esteban A, Anzueto A, Alía I, et al. How is mechanical ventilation employed in the intensive care unit? An international utilization review. Am J Respir Crit Care Med 2000;161(5):1450–8.

[5] Esteban A, Anzueto A, Frutos F, et al. Characteristics and outcomes in adult patients receiving mechanical ventilation: a 28-day international study. JAMA 2002;287(3):345–55.

[6] Dasta JF, McLaughlin TP, Mody SH, et al. Daily cost of an intensive care unit day: the contribution of mechanical ventilation. Crit Care Med 2005; 33(6):1266–71.

[7] Kress JP, Pohlman AS, O'Connor MF, et al. Daily interruption of sedative infusions in critically ill patients undergoing mechanical ventilation. N Engl J Med 2000;342:1471–7.

[8] Arroliga A, Frutos-Vivar F, Hall J, et al. Use of sedatives and neuromuscular blockers in a cohort of patients receiving mechanical ventilation. Chest 2005;128(2):496–506.

[9] Ostermann ME, Keenan SP, Seiferling RA, et al. Sedation in the intensive care unit: a systematic review. JAMA 2000;283(11):1451–9.

[10] Kress JP, Gehlbach B, Lacy M, et al. The long-term phsychological effects of daily sedative interruption on critically ill patients. Am J Respir Crit Care Med 2003;168:1457–61.

[11] Thille AW, Rodriguez P, Cabello B, et al. Patient-ventilator asynchrony during assisted mechanical ventilation. Intensive Care Med 2006;32(10): 1515–22.

[12] Chao DC, Scheinhorn DJ, Stearn-Hassenpflug M. Patient-ventilator trigger asynchrony in prolonged mechanical ventilation. Chest 1997;112(6):1592–9.

[13] Bosma K, Ferreyra G, Ambrogio C, et al. Patient-ventilator interaction and sleep in mechanically ventilated patients: pressure support versus proportional assist ventilation. Crit Care Med 2007;35(4): 1048–54.

[14] Greenough A, Milner AD, Dimitriou G. Synchronized mechanical ventilation for respiratory support in newborn infants. Cochrane Database Syst Rev 2004;(4):CD000456. Update of: Cochrane Database Syst Rev 2001;(1):CD000456.

[15] Mitchell RA, Berger AJ. Neural regulation of respiration. Am Rev Respir Dis 1975;111(2):206–24.

[16] Morélot-Panzini C, Fournier E, Donzel-Raynaud C, et al. J Conduction velocity of th ehuman phrenic nerve in the neck. Electromyogr Kinesiol 2007 [Epub ahead of print].

[17] Beck J, Sinderby C, Lindström L, et al. Effects of lung volume on diaphragm EMG signal strength during voluntary contractions. J Appl Physiol 1998;85(3):1123–34.

[18] Mier A, Brophy C, Moxham J, et al. Phrenic nerve stimulation in normal subjects and in patients with diaphragmatic weakness. Thorax 1987;42(11):885–8.

[19] McKenzie DK, Gandevia SC. Phrenic nerve conduction times and twitch pressures of the human diaphragm. J Appl Physiol 1985;58(5):1496–504.

[20] Beck J, Sinderby C, Lindström L, et al. Effects of chest wall configuration on diaphragm interference pattern EMG and compound muscle action potentials. J Appl Physiol 1997;82:520–30.

[21] Marini JJ. Dynamic hyperinflation. In: Marini JJ, Slutsky AS, editors. Lung biology in health and disease, vol. 118. Physiological basis of ventilatory support. New York: Marcel Dekker; 1998. p. 453–90.

[22] Hering E, Breuer J. Die Selbststeurung der athmung durch den nervus vagus. Sitzber Deut Akad Wiss Wein 1868;57:672–7.

[23] Widdicombe J. Airway receptors. Respir Physiol 2001;125(1–2):3–15.

[24] Widdicombe J. Reflexes from the lungs and airways: historical perspective. J Appl Physiol 2006; 101(2):628–34.

[25] Undem BJ, Kollarik M. The role of vagal afferent nerves in chronic obstructive pulmonary disease. Proc Am Thorac Soc 2005;2(4):355–60.

[26] Bailey EF, Fregosi RF. Modulation of upper airway muscle activities by bronchopulmonary afferents. J Appl Physiol 2006;101(2):609–17.

[27] Duron B, Jung-Caillol MC, Marlot D. Myelinated nerve fiber supply and muscle spindles in the respiratory muscles of cat: quantitative study. Anat Embryol (Berl) 1978;152(2):171–92.

[28] Jammes Y, Arbogast S, De Troyer A. Response of the rabbit diaphragm to tendon vibration. Neurosci Lett 2000;290(2):85–8.

[29] Corda M, Von Euler C, Lennerstrand G. Proprioceptive innervation of the diaphragm. J Physiol 1965;178:161–77.

[30] Cheeseman M, Revelette WR. Phrenic afferent contribution to reflexes elicited by changes in diaphragm length. J Appl Physiol 1990;69(2):640–7.

[31] Macron JM, Marlot D, Wallois F, et al. Phrenic-to-phrenic inhibition and excitation in spinal cats. Neurosci Lett 1988;91(1):24–9.

[32] Ward ME, Deschamps A, Roussos C, et al. Effect of phrenic afferent stimulation on pattern of respiratory muscle activation. J Appl Physiol 1992; 73(2):563–70.

[33] Supinski GS, Dick T, Stofan D, et al. Effects of intraphrenic injection of potassium on diaphragm activation. J Appl Physiol 1993;74(3):1186–94.

[34] De Troyer AD. The canine phrenic-to-intercostal reflex. J Physiol 1998;508(Pt 3):919–27.

[35] Butler JE, McKenzie DK, Gandevia SC. Reflex inhibition of human inspiratory muscles in response to contralateral phrenic nerve stimulation. Respir Physiol Neurobiol 2003;138(1):87–96.

[36] De Troyer A. Role of joint receptors in modulation of inspiratory intercostal activity by rib motion in dogs. J Physiol 1997;503(Pt 2):445–53.

[37] Frazier DT, Revelette WR. Role of phrenic nerve afferents in the control of breathing. J Appl Physiol 1991;70(2):491–6.

[38] Gourine AV. On the peripheral and central chemoreception and control of breathing: an emerging role of ATP. J Physiol 2005;568(Pt 3):715–24.

[39] Kara T, Narkiewicz K, Somers VK. Chemoreflexes—physiology and clinical implications. Acta Physiol Scand 2003;177(3):377–84.

[40] Nilsestuen JO, Hargett KD. Using ventilator graphics to identify patient-ventilator asynchrony. Respir Care 2005;50(2):202–34 [discussion: 232–4].

[41] Mulqueeny Q, Ceriana P, Carlucci A, et al. Automatic detection of ineffective triggering and double triggering during mechanical ventilation. Intensive Care Med 2007;33(11):2014–8.

[42] Younes M, Brochard L, Grasso S, et al. A method for monitoring and improving patient:ventilator interaction. Intensive Care Med 2007;33(8): 1337–46.

[43] Beck J, Campoccia F, Allo JC, et al. Improved synchrony and respiratory unloading by neurally adjusted ventilatory assist (NAVA) in lung-injured rabbits. Pediatr Res 2007;61(3):289–94.

[44] Leung P, Jubran A, Tobin MJ. Comparison of assisted ventilator modes on triggering, patient effort, and dyspnea. Am J Respir Crit Care Med 1997;155(6):1940–8.

[45] Aslanian P, El Atrous S, Isabey D, et al. Effects of flow triggering on breathing effort during partial ventilatory support. Am J Respir Crit Care Med 1998;157(1):135–43.

[46] Raux M, Ray P, Prella M, et al. Cerebral cortex activation during experimentally induced ventilator fighting in normal humans receiving noninvasive mechanical ventilation. Anesthesiology 2007; 107(5):746–55.

[47] Beck J, Gottfried SB, Navalesi P, et al. Electrical activity of the diaphragm during pressure support ventilation in acute respiratory failure. Am J Respir Crit Care Med 2001;164(3):419–24.

[48] Beck J, Weinberg J, Hamnegård CH, et al. Diaphragmatic function in advanced Duchenne muscular dystrophy. Neuromuscul Disord 2006; 16(3):161–7.

[49] Sinderby C, Beck J, Spahija J, et al. Voluntary activation of the human diaphragm in health and disease. J Appl Physiol 1998;85(6):2146–58.

[50] Barrera R, Melendez J, Ahdoot M, et al. Flow triggering added to pressure support ventilation improves comfort and reduces work of breathing in mechanically ventilated patients. J Crit Care 1999; 14(4):172–6.

[51] Parthasarathy S, Jubran A, Laghi F, et al. Sternomastoid, rib cage, and expiratory muscle activity during weaning failure. J Appl Physiol 2007; 103(1):140–7.

[52] Yan S, Sinderby C, Bielen P, et al. Expiratory muscle pressure and breathing mechanics in chronic obstructive pulmonary disease. Eur Respir J 2000; 16(4):684–90.

[53] Nava S, Bruschi C, Rubini F, et al. Respiratory response and inspiratory effort during pressure support ventilation in COPD patients. Intensive Care Med 1995;21(11):871–9.

[54] Appendini L, Purro A, Patessio A, et al. Partitioning of inspiratory muscle workload and pressure assistance in ventilator-dependent COPD patients. Am J Respir Crit Care Med 1996;154(5):1301–9.

[55] Sinderby C, Spahija J, Beck J, et al. Diaphragm activation during exercise in chronic obstructive pulmonary disease. Am J Respir Crit Care Med 2001;163(7):1637–41.

[56] Appendini L, Purro A, Gudjonsdottir M, et al. Physiologic response of ventilator-dependent patients with chronic obstructive pulmonary disease to proportional assist ventilation and continuous positive airway pressure. Am J Respir Crit Care Med 1999;159(5 Pt 1):1510–7.

[57] Imanaka H, Nishimura M, Takeuchi M, et al. Autotriggering caused by cardiogenic oscillation during flow-triggered mechanical ventilation. Crit Care Med 2000;28(2):402–7.

[58] Calderini E, Confalonieri M, Puccio PG, et al. Patient-ventilator asynchrony during noninvasive ventilation: the role of expiratory trigger. Intensive Care Med 1999;25(7):662–7.

[59] Beck J, Brander L, Slutsky AS, et al. Non-invasive neurally adjusted ventilatory assist in rabbits with acute lung injury. Intensive Care Med 2008;34: 316–23.

[60] Simon PM, Zurob AS, Wies WM, et al. Entrainment of respiration in humans by periodic lung inflations. Effect of state and CO(2). Am J Respir Crit Care Med 1999;160(3):950–60.

[61] MacDonald SM, Song G, Poon CS. Non-associative learning promotes respiratory entrainment to mechanical ventilation. PLoS ONE 2007;2(9): e865.

[62] Greenough A, Morley CJ, Pool J. Fighting the ventilator—are fast rates an effective alternative to paralysis? Early Hum Dev 1986;13(2):189–94.

[63] Yamada Y, Du HL. Analysis of the mechanisms of expiratory asynchrony in pressure support ventilation: a mathematical approach. J Appl Physiol 2000;88(6):2143–50.

[64] Kondili E, Prinianakis G, Anastasaki M, et al. Acute effects of ventilator settings on respiratory motor output in patients with acute lung injury. Intensive Care Med 2001;27:1147–57.

[65] Passam F, Hoing S, Prinianakis G, et al. Effect of different levels of pressure support and proportional assist ventilation on breathing pattern, work of breathing and gas exchange in mechanically ventilated hypercapnic COPD patients with acute respiratory failure. Respiration 2003;70(4): 355–61.

[66] Tokioka H, Tanaka T, Ishizu T, et al. The effect of breath termination criterion on breathing patterns and the work of breathing during pressure support ventilation. Anesth Analg 2001;92:161–5.

[67] Tassaux D, Gainnier M, Battisti A, et al. Impact of expiratory trigger setting on delayed cycling and inspiratory muscle workload. Am J Respir Crit Care Med 2005;172:1283–9.

[68] Chiumello D, Polli F, Tallarini F, et al. Effect of different cycling off criteria and positive end-expiratory pressure during pressure support ventilation in patients with chronic obstructive pulmonary disease. Crit Care Med 2007;35:2547–52.

[69] Younes M, Kun J, Webster K, et al. Response of ventilator-dependent patients to delayed opening of exhalation valve. Am J Respir Crit Care Med 2002;166:21–30.

[70] Beck J, Tucci M, Emeriaud G, et al. Prolonged neural expiratory time induced by mechanical ventilation in infants. Pediatr Res 2004;55:747–54.

[71] Giannouli E, Webster K, Roberts D, et al. Response of ventilator-dependent patients to different levels of pressure support and proportional assist. Am J Respir Crit Care Med 1999;159(6): 1716–25.

[72] Du HL, Ohtsuji M, Shigeta M, et al. Expiratory asynchrony in proportional assist ventilation. Am J Respir Crit Care Med 2002;165(7):972–7.

[73] Tobert DG, Simon PM, Stroetz RW, et al. The determinants of respiratory rate during mechanical ventilation. Am J Respir Crit Care Med 1997;155: 485–92.

[74] Georgopoulos D, Mitrouska I, Bshouty Z, et al. Effects of non-REM sleep on the response of respiratory output to varying inspiratory flow. Am J Respir Crit Care Med 1996;153:1624–30.

[75] Corne S, Webster K, Younes M. Effects of inspiratory flow on diaphragmatic motor output in normal subjects. J Appl Physiol 2000;89:481–92.

[76] Fernandez R, Mendez M, Younes M. Effect of ventilator flow rate on respiratory timing in normal humans. Am J Respir Crit Care Med 1999;159: 710–9.

[77] Laghi F, Segal J, Choe WK, et al. Effect of imposed inflation time on respiratory frequency and hyperinflation in patients with chronic obstructive pulmonary disease. Am J Respir Crit Care Med 2001;163(6):1365–70.

[78] Puddy A, Younes M. Effect of slowly increasing elastic load on breathing in conscious humans. J Appl Physiol 1991;70(3):1277–83.

[79] Chiumello D, Pelosi P, Taccone P, et al. Effect of different inspiratory rise time and cycling off criteria during pressure support ventilation in patients recovering from acute lung injury. Crit Care Med 2003;31(11):2604–10.

[80] Jaecklin T, Morel DR, Rimensberger PC. Volume-targeted modes of modern neonatal ventilators: how stable is the delivered tidal volume? Intensive Care Med 2007;33(2):326–35, Epub 2006 Nov 22.

[81] Scopesi F, Calevo MG, Rolfe P, et al. Volume targeted ventilation (volume guarantee) in the weaning phase of premature newborn infants. Pediatr Pulmonol 2007;42(10):864–70.

[82] van Kaam AH, Rimensberger PC. Lung-protective ventilation strategies in neonatology: what do we know–what do we need to know? Crit Care Med 2007;35(3):925–31.

[83] Brunner JX, Iotti GA. Adaptive support ventilation (ASV). Minerva Anestesiol 2002;68(5):365–8.

[84] Arnal JM, Wysocki M, Nafati C, et al. Automatic selection of breathing pattern using adaptive support ventilation. Intensive Care Med 2008;34: 75–81.

[85] Dojat M, Brochard L, Lemaire F, et al. A knowledge-based system for assisted ventilation of patients in intensive care units. Int J Clin Monit Comput 1992;9:239–50.

[86] Lellouche F, Mancebo J, Jolliet P, et al. A multicenter randomized trial of computer-driven protocolized weaning from mechanical ventilation. Am J Respir Crit Care Med 2006;174(8):894–900.

[87] Nava S, Bruschi C, Fracchia C, et al. Patient-ventilator interaction and inspiratory effort during pressure support ventilation in patients with different pathologies. Eur Respir J 1997;10(1): 177–83.

[88] Allo JC, Beck JC, Brander L, et al. Influence of neurally adjusted ventilatory assist and positive end-expiratory pressure on breathing pattern in rabbits with acute lung injury. Crit Care Med 2006;34:2997–3004.

[89] Brander L, Leong-Poi H, Hansen MS, et al. Neurally adjusted ventilatory assist (NAVA) in patients with hypoxic respiratory failure. Intensive Care Med 2006;32(S13):S119 (abstract).

[90] Spahija J, de Marchie M, Bellemare P, et al. Patient-ventilator interaction during pressure support ventilation (PSV) and neurally adjusted ventilatory assist (NAVA) in acute respiratory failure (abstract). Proceedings of the ATS 2005;A847.

[91] Marantz S, Patrick W, Webster K, et al. Response of ventilator-dependent patients to different levels of proportional assist. J Appl Physiol 1996;80(2): 397–403.

[92] Meza S, Giannouli E, Younes M. Control of breathing during sleep assessed by proportional assist ventilation. J Appl Physiol 1998;84(1):3–12.

[93] Pankow W, Penzel T, Juhasz J, et al. Influence of proportional assist ventilation on diaphragmatic activity in normal subjects. Eur J Med Res 2004; 9(10):461–7.

[94] Delaere S, Roeseler J, D'hoore W, et al. Respiratory muscle workload in intubated, spontaneously breathing patients without COPD: pressure support vs proportional assist ventilation. Intensive Care Med 2003;29(6):949–54.

[95] Navalesi P, Hernandez P, Wongsa A, et al. Proportional assist ventilation in acute respiratory failure: effects on breathing pattern and inspiratory effort. Am J Respir Crit Care Med 1996;154(5):1330–8.

[96] Wysocki M, Meshaka P, Richard JC, et al. Proportional-assist ventilation compared with pressure-support ventilation during exercise in volunteers with external thoracic restriction. Crit Care Med 2004;32(2):409–14.

[97] Grasso S, Puntillo F, Mascia L, et al. Compensation for increase in respiratory workload during mechanical ventilation. Pressure-support versus proportional-assist ventilation. Am J Respir Crit Care Med 2000;161(3 Pt 1):819–26.

[98] Ranieri VM, Giuliani R, Mascia L, et al. Patient-ventilator interaction during acute hypercapnia: pressure-support vs. proportional-assist ventilation. J Appl Physiol 1996;81(1):426–36.

[99] Kondili E, Xirouchaki N, Vaporidi K, et al. Short-term cardiorespiratory effects of proportional assist and pressure-support ventilation in patients with acute lung injury/acute respiratory distress syndrome. Anesthesiology 2006;105(4):703–8.

[100] Varelmann D, Wrigge H, Zinserling J, et al. Proportional assist versus pressure support ventilation in patients with acute respiratory failure:

cardiorespiratory responses to artificially increased ventilatory demand. Crit Care Med 2005;33(9): 1968–75.

[101] Schulze A, Rieger-Fackeldey E, Gerhardt T, et al. Randomized crossover comparison of proportional assist ventilation and patient-triggered ventilation in extremely low birth weight infants with evolving chronic lung disease. Neonatology 2007; 92(1):1–7.

[102] Schulze A, Gerhardt T, Musante G, et al. Proportional assist ventilation in low birth weight infants with acute respiratory disease: a comparison to assist/control and conventional mechanical ventilation. J Pediatr 1999;135(3):339–44.

[103] Rieger-Fackeldey E, Schaller-Bals S, Schulze A. Effect of body temperature on the pattern of spontaneous breathing in extremely low birth weight infants supported by proportional assist ventilation. Pediatr Res 2003;54(3):332–6 E.

[104] Ye Q, Wang C, Tong Z, et al. Proportional assist ventilation: methodology and therapeutics on COPD patients compared with pressure support ventilation. Chin Med J (Engl) 2002;115(2):179–83.

[105] Fang Z, Niu S, Zhu L, et al. Distribution of ventilation and hemodynamic effects of different ventilatory patterns. Chin Med J (Engl) 2002;115(2): 188–91.

[106] Mitrouska J, Xirouchaki N, Patakas D, et al. Effects of chemical feedback on respiratory motor and ventilatory output during different modes of assisted mechanical ventilation. Eur Respir J 1999;13(4):873–82.

[107] Wrigge H, Golisch W, Zinserling J, et al. Proportional assist versus pressure support ventilation: effects on breathing pattern and respiratory work of patients with chronic obstructive pulmonary disease. Intensive Care Med 1999;25(8):790–8.

[108] Leipälä JA, Iwasaki S, Lee S, et al. Compliance and resistance levels and unloading in proportional assist ventilation. Physiol Meas 2005;26(3):281–92.

[109] Younes M, Webster K, Kun J, et al. A method for measuring passive elastance during proportional assist ventilation. Am J Respir Crit Care Med 2001;164(1):50–60.

[110] Younes M, Kun J, Masiowski B, et al. A method for noninvasive determination of inspiratory resistance during proportional assist ventilation. Am J Respir Crit Care Med 2001;163(4):829–39.

[111] Kondili E, Prinianakis G, Alexopoulou C, et al. Respiratory load compensation during mechanical ventilation–proportional assist ventilation with load-adjustable gain factors versus pressure support. Intensive Care Med 2006;32(5):692–9.

[112] Wysocki M, Richard JC, Meshaka P. Noninvasive proportional assist ventilation compared with noninvasive pressure support ventilation in hypercapnic acute respiratory failure. Crit Care Med 2002;30(2):323–9.

[113] Vitacca M, Clini E, Pagani M, et al. Physiologic effects of early administered mask proportional assist ventilation in patients with chronic obstructive pulmonary disease and acute respiratory failure. Crit Care Med 2000;28(6):1791–7.

[114] Winck JC, Vitacca M, Morais A, et al. Tolerance and physiologic effects of nocturnal mask pressure support vs proportional assist ventilation in chronic ventilatory failure. Chest 2004;126(2):382–8.

[115] Fernández-Vivas M, Caturla-Such J, González de la Rosa J, et al. Noninvasive pressure support versus proportional assist ventilation in acute respiratory failure. Intensive Care Med 2003;29(7):1126–33.

[116] Porta R, Appendini L, Vitacca M, et al. Mask proportional assist vs pressure support ventilation in patients in clinically stable condition with chronic ventilatory failure. Chest 2002;122(2):479–88.

[117] Serra A, Polese G, Braggion C, et al. Non-invasive proportional assist and pressure support ventilation in patients with cystic fibrosis and chronic respiratory failure. Thorax 2002;57(1):50–4.

[118] Gay PC, Hess DR, Hill NS. Noninvasive proportional assist ventilation for acute respiratory insufficiency. Comparison with pressure support ventilation. Am J Respir Crit Care Med 2001; 164(9):1606–11.

[119] Sinderby C, Beck J, Spahija J, et al. Inspiratory muscle unloading by neurally adjusted ventilatory assist during maximal inspiratory efforts in healthy subjects. Chest 2007;131(3):711–7.

[120] The Acute Respiratory Distress Syndrome Network. Ventilation with lower tidal volumes as compared with traditional tidal volumes for acute lung injury and the acute respiratory distress syndrome. N Engl J Med 2000;342:1301–8.

[121] Jubran A, Van de Graaff WB, Tobin MJ. Variability of patient-ventilator interaction with pressure support ventilation in patients with chronic obstructive pulmonary disease. Am J Respir Crit Care Med 1995;152(1):129–36.

[122] Parthasarathy S, Jubran A, Tobin MJ. Cycling of inspiratory and expiratory muscle groups with the ventilator in airflow limitation. Am J Respir Crit Care Med 1998;158(5 Pt 1):1471–8.

ELSEVIER
SAUNDERS

Clin Chest Med 29 (2008) 343–350

CLINICS
IN CHEST
MEDICINE

Does Closed Loop Control of Assist Control Ventilation Reduce Ventilator-Induced Lung Injury?

Richard D. Branson, MSc, RRT*, Kenneth Davis, Jr, MD

University of Cincinnati, 231 Albert Sabin Way, Cincinnati, OH 45267-0558, USA

Conventional mechanical ventilation is commonly accomplished using either a constant volume or constant pressure breath [1]. It is an important distinction that the breath type is separate from the mode of ventilation. The mode of ventilation describes the ventilator response to patient effort and control of phase variables. As such, pressure or volume breaths can be delivered in the continuous mandatory ventilation or intermittent mandatory ventilation (IMV) mode. Volume-controlled breaths are delivered using a peak inspiratory flow set by the clinician and an inspiratory flow waveform (commonly rectangular) determined by the ventilator. Delivered tidal volume is constant as long as no alarm settings are violated. Airway pressure is variable based on patient effort, respiratory system compliance, and airway resistance. Specifically, with greater patient effort, airway pressure falls. As compliance falls or resistance increases, peak airway pressure increases and vice versa.

Pressure controlled breaths do not have a set peak flow or flow waveform. The flow is controlled by the ventilator and varies breath to breath to achieve the preset pressure limit. For a passive inspiration, the flow waveform is an exponential decay (often referred to as decelerating) and peak flow depends on respiratory system compliance and resistance. For an active inspiration, flow is highly irregular, depending on the patient's inspiratory effort. Airway pressure is constant and delivered tidal volume is a function of patient effort, respiratory system compliance, and airway resistance. When compliance is low or resistance is high, the flow during pressure controlled breaths may reach zero and the remainder of inspiratory time is similar to an inspiratory pause.

A comparison of volume and pressure controlled breaths is outside the realm of this article, but this topic has been detailed elsewhere [2]. However, it is important to summarize these differences, to understand the thought process behind a type of "self adjusting" breath control that attempts to achieve the best features of volume and pressure control. Volume control allows a guarantee of tidal volume and minute volume. These attributes may be particularly helpful in a patient with varying pulmonary compliance, hypercarbia, and in the implementation of a lung protective approach. However, the fixed flow of volume control can lead to flow dys-synchrony and excessive work of breathing. Pressure control limits the maximum airway pressure seen by the lung, while reducing work of breathing as a virtue of the variable flow and flow waveform. Pressure control then might reduce ventilator-induced lung injury (VILI), reduce work of breathing, and enhance patient ventilator synchrony in the active patient. However, during pressure control ventilation, the tidal volume is variable and both hyperventilation and hypoventilation are possible. Adaptive pressure control attempts to improve patient synchrony by allowing as much flow as the patient demands, while also attempting to guarantee a minimum tidal volume [3,4]. This is a critical point of understanding: adaptive pressure control does not prevent the tidal volume from being greater than the set tidal volume, it simply prevents it from falling below the preset volume.

* Corresponding author. Division of Trauma/Critical Care, University of Cincinnati Medical Center, 231 Bethesda Avenue, Cincinnati, OH 45207-0558.

E-mail address: richard.branson@uc.edu (R.D. Branson).

Definition of adaptive pressure control

During adaptive pressure control, inspiration is machine or patient triggered, pressure limited, and machine or patient cycled. The breathing pattern can be continuous mandatory ventilation, intermittent mandatory ventilation, or continuous spontaneous ventilation (pressure support). The unique aspect of adaptive pressure control is that the pressure limit is not constant, but varies from one breath to the next based on a comparison of the set and delivered inspiratory tidal volume. The logic for controlling the output of the current breath based on the previous breath has led this technique to be called "dual control, breath to breath" [4–10]. It is important to remember that the ventilator can only control pressure or volume during a single breath, not both. So adaptive pressure control is a pressure controlled inspiration with a volume target: that is, it is called a target because unlike volume control the tidal volume may be higher or lower than planned, in which case an alert may be activated. Adaptive pressure control is provided by a number of ventilators using a variety of names.

While there are some subtle differences in the algorithms that control these techniques, operation is fairly similar. Upon selecting a mode with adaptive pressure control, the ventilator provides a test breath. This test breath can be at a constant pressure or volume. The test breath allows the total respiratory system compliance to be measured. The algorithm can then calculate the pressure required to deliver the tidal volume set by the clinician. The ventilator may initially deliver 75% to 100% of the calculated pressure. The tidal volume leaving the ventilator (note, this is not exhaled tidal volume) is then compared with the tidal volume set and the pressure on the subsequent breath is either held constant (if the set tidal volume is met) or adjusted (increased if the tidal volume is greater than set, decreased if tidal volume is less than set). Most ventilators limit the maximum change from one breath to the next at 3 cm H_2O. The minimum inspiratory pressure is typically positive end-expiratory pressure (PEEP) plus 5 cm H_2O, and the maximum inspiratory pressure is the high pressure alarm setting minus 5 cm H_2O or 10 cm H_2O. If the set tidal volume cannot be delivered because of the high-pressure setting, an alert is generated. This alert typically provides a message, such as "volume not constant" or "check pressure limit," such that the clinician is aware that the desired tidal volume is not being delivered.

Adaptive support ventilation

Adaptive support ventilation (ASV) is a rule-based mode of ventilation that guides the patient to achieve a minimum minute ventilation (V_E) using what is touted as an optimal breathing pattern. ASV uses "hard" and "soft" rules based on respiratory mechanics. Hard rules are preset limits that are not affected by user input or patient characteristics. Soft rules are determined by clinician input and measured patient characteristics and may change over time. The clinician determines the minimum (target) V_E by input of the patient's ideal body weight (IBW) and setting a control referred to as "% Minute Volume" (% Min Vol). IBW may range from 10 kg to 200 kg and should be calculated using the following formulas [3]:

$$IBW = 50 + 2.3$$
$$(\text{Height in inches} - 60) \text{ for males,}$$

and

$$IBW = 45.5 + 2.3$$
$$(\text{Height in inches} - 60) \text{ for females}$$

IBW is used according to the Radford nomogram to determine the anatomic dead space of the patient at 2.2 mL/kg [4]. IBW is also used to determine two soft rule boundaries for high and low tidal volume (V_T) at 15.4 and 4.4 times IBW, respectively. The lower boundary assures the minimum V_T will be two times dead space (V_D).

Once the IBW is entered, target V_E is determined by the % Min Vol control according to the following formulas:

$$V_E \text{ target} = 100 * \% \text{ Min Vol}$$
$$* IBW (\text{for IBW} > 15 \text{kg}),$$

or

$$V_E \text{ target} = 200 * \% \text{ Min Vol}$$
$$* IBW (\text{for IBW} < 5 \text{kg})$$

The % Min Vol control is adjustable from 25% to 350% to account for variations in alveolar dead space caused by ventilation or perfusion mismatch and changes in carbon dioxide production. An adult patient with an IBW of 75 kg set to 100% Min Vol will have a target V_E of 7.5 L per minute. The % Min Vol setting determines a soft boundary for high mandatory breath rate based on the following formulas:

Max. f = 22bpm

   $* \%$ Min Vol/100 (if IBW $>$ 15kg),

or

Max. f = 45bpm

   $* \%$ Min Vol/100 (if IBW $<$ 15kg)

The hard boundaries for mandatory breath rate are a minimum of 5 beats per minute (bpm) and a maximum of 60 bpm. Because the minimum mandatory breath rate is 5 bpm, a soft boundary for maximum mandatory V_T is dependant on the target V_E (ie, Max V_T = target V_E/5).

The ASV algorithm will determine the optimal breathing pattern (f and V_T) by applying the "minimum work of breathing" concept, described by Otis and colleagues in 1950 [11]. This concept suggests the patient will breathe at a V_T and frequency combination that will minimize the cumulative effects of elastic and resistive loads imposed on and by the respiratory system. The following equation describes patient selection of optimal respiratory rate using Otis' minimal work concept:

$$RR = \sqrt{[1 + 4\pi^2 RCe \cdot (V_A/V_D) - 1]/2\pi^2 RCe}$$

Where RR is respiratory rate, RCe is expiratory time constant (product of airways resistance and respiratory system compliance), V_A is alveolar ventilation, and V_D is dead space volume. For example, a 75-kg patient with a respiratory system compliance of 0.05 L/cm H_2O, airway resistance of 5 cm H_2O/L/sec, and an added resistance of 5 cm H_2O/L/sec (because of the exhalation valve and breathing circuit) would have a calculated RCe of 0.5 seconds (0.05 L/cm H_2O × 10 cm H_2O/L/sec). With the % Min Vol set to 100%, the target V_E is 7.5 L per minute.

If no patient effort is detected, the target breathing pattern will be imposed on the patient using mandatory breaths that are pressure limited, volume targeted, and time cycled (adaptive pressure control breaths). The inspiratory pressure of each mandatory breath is determined by the pressure to volume relationship measured during the previous eight breaths. Inspiratory pressure may be adjusted by up to 2 cm H_2O per breath to deliver the target V_T. The minimum inspiratory

pressure is 5 cm H_2O above baseline. The maximum inspiratory pressure is determined by the clinician's setting of the high pressure limit alarm (P_{max}). The P_{max} is the pressure at which an alarm (airway pressure high) will sound and inspiration will be terminated. The ASV controller, however, will not target a pressure within 10 cm H_2O of the P_{max} (ie, if the P_{max} is set to 45 cm H_2O, the highest target pressure during ASV is 35 cm H_2O). In this case, an alarm (unable to reach target) will sound if the target V_T is not achieved.

Inspiratory time and inspiratory to expiratory (I:E) ratio during mandatory breath delivery are controlled by the ASV algorithm and are determined by calculations including rate, V_E, V_D, and RCe. The ASV rule base also sets boundaries for inspiratory and expiratory time. Hard rules for the minimum and maximum inspiratory time are 0.5 and 2 seconds, respectively. In addition, the minimum inspiratory time must be greater than or equal to 1 RCe. Minimum expiratory time is equal to 3 RCe, which should allow exhalation of at least 95% of the inspired volume [12]. This rule may also affect the maximum breath rate according to the following formula: $f_{max} = 15/RCe$. These timing limitations are imposed to avoid rapid breath rates, which may result in gas trapping, high dead space ventilation, and the development of intrinsic PEEP. The maximum expiratory time is 15 seconds and the limits for I:E ratio are 1:4 to 1:1.

In the event that patient breathing effort is detected, ASV will deliver breaths that are pressure limited, volume targeted, and flow cycled (ie, adaptive pressure, pressure support). As patient contribution to the target V_E increases, the ASV algorithm will automatically reduce the mandatory breath rate. ASV will continue to target an "optimal" breathing pattern, although during spontaneous breathing, the only parameter being controlled by ASV is inspiratory pressure. The patient may dictate breath rate, inspiratory and expiratory times, and V_E (as long as V_E exceeds the target V_E). The rule base of ASV remains in place and the patient is guided to the optimal breathing pattern solely by manipulation of inspiratory pressure.

Controls that must be set by the clinician during ASV include: PEEP, F_iO_2, rise time, expiratory trigger sensitivity, and inspiratory trigger sensitivity. The basic breath delivery during ASV is an adaptive pressure breath. However, ASV also allows automated control of respiratory rate and I:E, a feature which is not part of the typical adaptive pressure control system.

Volume control versus pressure control versus adaptive pressure control versus adaptive support

The question posed here is, do these new breath types protect the patient from VILI or is it possible that VILI could be worsened? No studies have been accomplished in human beings or animals to answer this question adequately. Instead, the authors will look at the literature regarding the use of these techniques and specifically evaluate the tidal volume and airway pressures delivered.

While volume control provides a constant volume and variable airway pressure, and pressure control provides a constant airway pressure and variable tidal volume, the goal of adaptive pressure control is to provide a constant tidal volume at the lowest possible airway pressure. So while adaptive pressure control was designed to combine the positive attributes of both volume and pressure control, the response to changes in patient condition can result in a variable response with each breath type. Adaptive pressure control cannot guarantee a set tidal volume if the patient's respiratory system compliance is too low and the high pressure alarm is set too low. As an example, if the patients' lung compliance is 20 mL/cm H_2O, the desired tidal volume is 600 mL, and the P_{max} is 25 cm H_2O, the maximum tidal volume that can be delivered is 20 cm H_2O × 20 mL/cm H_2O = 400 mL. In this instance, an alert would be provided by the ventilator that the "tidal volume is not met." There is no magic to an adaptive pressure breath; the rules of gas movement still apply. Similarly, adaptive pressure control cannot limit the inspired tidal volume beyond reducing the peak airway pressure. If the patient can generate a tidal volume greater than the desired tidal volume, the volume will not be less than the desired volume but it can be greater. Table 1 lists characteristics of the four techniques and the response to common clinical conditions.

Literature review

There are no randomized controlled trials of modes using adaptive pressure control in large numbers of patients. In fact, the literature remains sparse with regard to the utility of this control scheme, although the same can be said for many new ventilator techniques and modes. This review then will concentrate on the findings of smaller trials and case series.

Piotrowski and colleagues [13] compared pressure regulated volume control (PRVC) (ie,

adaptive pressure controlled continuous mandatory ventilation) to volume controlled IMV in 60 neonates with respiratory distress syndrome using a randomized, prospective design. Thirty subjects received IMV and 27 received PRVC. All subjects suffered from either respiratory distress syndrome or congenital pneumonia and weighed less than 2,500 grams. They selected duration of mechanical ventilation and incidence of bronchopulmonary dysplasia as the main outcome variables. Secondary outcomes were complications including the incidence of air leaks, intraventricular hemorrhage (IVH), and hemodynamic instability. They did not show any differences in the main outcome variables. However, they reported a reduction in the incidence of IVH grade II and greater PRVC group. During data mining they found that in infants weighing less than 1,000 grams, the duration of ventilation was shorter and the incidence of hypotension was reduced with PRVC. However, this post-hoc analysis included only 10 subjects in each group.

Alvarez and colleagues [14] compared volume controlled ventilation (VCV), pressure-limited time-cycled ventilation, and PRVC in 10 adult subjects with acute respiratory failure and reported that PRVC resulted in a lower peak airway pressure and a slight improvement in carbon dioxide elimination compared with VCV. Subjects were ventilated using VCV with a constant inspiratory flow waveform, pressure control ventilation (PCV), and PRVC for 1 hour each. Not surprisingly, the peak inspiratory pressure was highest with the constant flow waveform, and there were no differences between PCV and PRVC.

Kesecioglu and colleagues [15–17] compared VCV and PRVC in a pig model of acute respiratory distress syndrome (ARDS) in a series of publications. These animal studies used short-term observational periods following saline lavage-induced ARDS. Their main findings were reduced airway pressures and small improvements in gas exchange compared with volume control ventilation with a constant inspiratory flow. In each of these studies, PRVC was delivered using an inverse I:E ratio.

Guldager and colleagues [18] compared VCV with a constant flow to PRVC in a prospective, open, cross over trial of 44 subjects with acute respiratory failure. Subjects were evaluated during an 8-hour stabilization period and then randomized to one mode or the other. After 2 hours, measurements were obtained and subjects switched to the other mode for 2 hours. At the end of this

Table 1
Characteristics of volume control, pressure control, adaptive pressure control, and adaptive support ventilation, and response to common clinical conditions

	Volume control	Pressure control	Adaptive pressure control	Adaptive support
Volume	Constant	Variable	Variable	Variable
Pressure	Variable	Constant	Variable	Variable
Flow	Constant	Variable	Variable	Variable
Flow Waveform	Constant	Variable	Variable	Variable
Response to common clinical conditions				
Decreased compliance	P_{aw}–increased V_T–constant	P_{aw}–constant V_T–decreased	P_{aw}–increased V_T–constant	P_{aw}–increased V_T–constant Or P_{aw}–constant V_T–decreased RR–increased
Increased compliance	P_{aw}–decreased V_T–constant	P_{aw}–constant V_T–increased	P_{aw}–decreased V_T–constant	P_{aw}–decreased V_T–constant Or P_{aw}–constant V_T–increased RR–decreased
Increased patient effort	P_{aw}–decreased V_T–constant	P_{aw}–constant V_T–increased	P_{aw}–decreased V_T–constant or greater than set	P_{aw}–decreased V_T–constant or greater than set Change from time cycled to flow cycled breaths
PEEPi	P_{aw}–increased V_T–constant	P_{aw}–constant V_T–decreased	P_{aw}–increased V_T–constant	P_{aw}–increased V_T–constant Or P_{aw}–constant or decreased V_T–decreased RR–increased T_I–decreased

Abbreviations: P_{aw}, airway pressure; PEEPi, intrinsic positive end-expiratory pressure; RR, respiratory rate; T_I, inspiratory time; V_T, tidal volume.

second period, measurements were obtained and the subject returned to the initial mode of ventilation for the duration of ventilatory support. During the short-term observations, blood gases, airway pressure, and mean arterial pressure were recorded. Long-term observations included duration of mechanical ventilation, days with a peak inspiratory pressure (PIP) greater than 50 cm H_2O, and survival. During ventilation with either mode, tidal volume was set at 5 mL/kg to 8 mL/kg and I:E of 1:3. PIP was significantly lower with PRVC (24 cm H_2O versus 20 cm H_2O), but plateau pressures were not recorded. All other short-term observational variables were not clinically or statistically different. Survival and duration of ventilation were similar. Two patients in the VCV group had a PIP greater than 50 cm H_2O compared with no patients in the PRVC

group. This was not statistically different, nor is it surprising because pressure can be limited during PRVC.

Kocis and colleagues [19] compared PRVC to VCV in infants after surgery for congenital heart disease. The infants were initially stabilized using VCV for 30 minutes. At the end of this period blood gases, hemodynamic, and ventilation parameters were recorded. The subjects were then placed on PRVC for 30 minutes and had the same data collected. This was followed by a second period of VCV. The only statistically significant change in any of the measured variables was a decrease in PIP of 19% during PRVC (31 cm H_2O to 25 cm H_2O). As in other studies, plateau pressures were not recorded.

Jaber and colleagues [20] recently evaluated volume support (VS, ie: adaptive pressure controlled continuous spontaneous ventilation) on the Siemens Servo 300 ventilator and pressure support during an increase in ventilatory demand. They added dead space to the ventilator circuit to cause rebreathing and stimulate ventilatory drive. This was not done using VS, but the mechanisms would be very similar. They found that with VS, rebreathing resulted in an increase in the work of breathing and pressure time product. During VS, the increases in the work of breathing and pressure time product were 2.5 to 4 times greater than during pressure support. The increase in patient effort resulted in a decrease in pressure during VS of 6 cm H_2O (15 cm H_2O to 9 cm H_2O). In two subjects, this resulted in "overt respiratory distress" according to the investigators.

Kallet and colleagues [21] compared VCV, PCV, and PRVC during implementation of a low tidal volume strategy in an effort to elucidate changes in the work of breathing. They found that while the pressure-controlled breaths could reduce the work of breathing, this was achieved by delivery of a larger tidal volume, exceeding the 6-mL/kg goal. When the pressure was reduced to achieve the tidal volume target, work of breathing was actually higher with the pressure-controlled breaths. This study begs some important questions regarding the choice of tidal volume and whether higher tidal volumes at low plateau pressures are safe. It also demonstrates the difficulty in comparing breath delivery techniques in an active patient population. It is possible that the variable tidal volume during pressure control, and the ability to exceed 6 mL/kg when airway pressures are less than 25 cm H_2O, might reduce the work of breathing while still providing lung protection.

The support for the use of adaptive pressure control confirms that PIP is lower when compared with VCV with a constant flow waveform. Studies have failed to show any advantage in reducing duration of ventilation, reducing complications, altering survival, or improving synchrony. The total number of subjects studied remains small at 133, with half being neonates and over a quarter, subjects without lung disease. The comparison of adaptive pressure control to VCV with a constant flow waveform and demonstration of a lower PIP is easily explained and predictable. The use of adaptive pressure control is quite popular for any number of reasons. However, similar effects can be accomplished with traditional pressure control ventilation or VCV using a descending ramp flow waveform [22].

ASV has been studied by a number of investigators. The majority of these studies evaluate the ability of ASV to choose initial ventilatory parameters or as a technique to facilitate weaning after cardiac surgery [23–29]. Two recent studies specifically evaluate the use of ASV in respiratory failure [30,31]. Both are observational trials evaluating the use of ASV with no comparator.

In the study by Arnal [31], tidal volume delivery was determined for subjects based on diagnostic category. This included subjects with normal lungs, chronic obstructive lung disease (COPD), acute lung injury (ALI), chest wall stiffness, and acute respiratory failure. Interestingly, the average PEEP in each of these groups was 5 cm H_2O to 8 cm H_2O, suggesting patients who were not particularly ill. Fig. 1 depicts the average tidal volume for each of the diagnostic categories in ml/kg from the Arnal study. During ALI, the tidal volume averaged 8.1 mL/kg, with a range of 6.7 mL/kg to 8.8 mL/kg. Peak inspiratory pressure averaged 28 cm H_2O, with a range of 23 cm H_2O to 33 cm H_2O. In the COPD population, tidal volumes as high as 9.5 mL/kg were delivered.

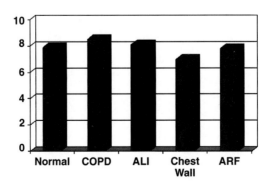

Fig. 1. The average tidal volume for each of the diagnostic categories in ml/kg from the Arnal study.

The investigators conclude that ASV is able to select the appropriate V_T and RR combinations for patients with variable respiratory mechanics. They do note that in actively breathing patients the tidal volume differences between diagnostic groups were less clear.

Summary

The issue at hand is whether or not adaptive pressure control or adaptive support ventilation can reduce VILI. Clearly, the answer based on the evidence is, we don't know. Understanding how these techniques work can allow us to speculate as to this issue. Neither pressure control nor adaptive pressure control limit the tidal volume delivery. It is possible in an active patient for tidal volumes to exceed 10 mL/kg, even though plateau pressures remain less than 30 cm H_2O. Whether this results in ALI or worsens ALI remains to be seen. ASV is simply adaptive pressure control with additional control over respiratory rate and I:E. Because the clinician can choose the absolute P_{max} in ASV, this technique may have an advantage over adaptive pressure control alone. When faced with a lower tidal volume constraint, ASV adjusts respiratory rate to preserve minute ventilation and I:E to prevent air-trapping. The major limitation of ASV is that when the patient is actively breathing, it is simply adaptive pressure support with only control over the peak pressure of each breath.

If the clinician desires to control tidal volume during mechanical ventilation for ALI, volume control ventilation is the only technique that provides that ability. During pressure ventilation of any kind, tidal volume can be greater than desired. The clinical implications of this finding are unclear.

References

[1] Branson RD, Chatburn RL. Classification of mechanical ventilators. In: MacIntyre NR, Branson RD, editors. Mechanical ventilation. Philadelphia: W.B. Saunders; 2000:1–33.

[2] Hess DR, Branson RD. New ventilator modes. In: Hill NH, Levy ML, editors. Ventilator management strategies for critical care. New York: Marcel Dekker; 2001. p. 172–223.

[3] Chatburn RL. Computer control of mechanical ventilation. Respir Care 2004;49(5):507–15.

[4] Chatburn RL. Classification of ventilator modes: update and proposal for implementation. Respir Care 2007;52(3):301–23.

[5] Branson RD. Techniques for automated feedback control of mechanical ventilation. Semin Respir Crit Care Med 2000;21:203–10.

[6] Hess DR, Branson RD. Ventilators and weaning modes. Respir Care Clin N Am 2000;6:193–225.

[7] Branson RD, Campbell RS, Davis K, et al. Closed loop ventilation. Respir Care 2002;47:427–53.

[8] Branson RD, Davis K Jr. Dual control modes. Respir Care Clin N Am 2001;7(3):397–408.

[9] Branson RD, MacIntyre NR. Dual-control modes of mechanical ventilation. Respir Care 1996;41: 294–305.

[10] Branson RD, Johannigman JA. What is the evidence base for the newer ventilation modes? Respir Care 2004;49(7):742–60.

[11] Otis AB, Fenn WO, Rahn H. Mechanics of breathing in man. J Appl Physiol 1950;2:592–607.

[12] Brunner JX, Laubscher TP, Banner MJ, et al. A simple method to measure total expiratory time constant based on the passive expiratory flow-volume curve. Crit Care Med 1995;23:1117–22.

[13] Piotrowski A, Sobala W, Kawczynski P. Patient initiated, pressure regulated, volume controlled ventilation compared with intermittent mandatory ventilation in neonates: a prospective, randomised study. Intensive Care Med 1997;23:975–81.

[14] Alvarez A, Subirana M, Benito S. Decelerating flow ventilation effects in acute respiratory failure. J Crit Care 1998;13:21–5.

[15] Kesecioglu J, Telci L, Tutuncu AS, et al. Effects of volume controlled ventilation with PEEP, pressure regulated volume controlled ventilation and low frequency positive pressure ventilation with extracorporeal carbon dioxide removal on total static lung compliance and oxygenation in pigs with ARDS. Adv Exp Med Biol 1996;388:629–36.

[16] Kesecioglu J, Gultuna I, Pompe JC, et al. Assessment of ventilation inhomogeneity and gas exchange with volume controlled ventilation and pressure regulated volume controlled ventilation on pigs with surfactant depleted lungs. Adv Exp Med Biol 1996;388:539–44.

[17] Kesecioglu J, Telci L, Esen F, et al. Respiratory and haemodynamic effects of conventional volume controlled PEEP, pressure regulated volume controlled ventilation ventilation and low frequency positive pressure ventilation with extracorporeal carbon dioxide removal in pigs with acute ARDS. Acta Anaesthesiol Scand 1994;38:879–84.

[18] Guldager H, Nielsen SL, Carl P, et al. A comparison of volume control ventilation and pressure regulated volume control ventilation in acute respiratory failure. Crit Care 1997;1:75–7.

[19] Kocis KC, Dekeon MK, Rosen HK, et al. Pressure regulated volume control vs volume control ventilation in infants after surgery for congenital heart disease. Pediatr Cardiol 2001;22:233–7.

[20] Jaber S, Delay JM, Matecki S, et al. Volume-guaranteed pressure-support ventilation facing

acute changes in ventilatory demand. Intensive Care
Med 2005;31(9):1181–8.

[21] Kallet RH, Campbell AR, Dicker RA, et al. Work of
breathing during lung-protective ventilation in
patients with acute lung injury and acute respiratory
distress syndrome: a comparison between volume
and pressure-regulated breathing modes. Respir
Care 2005;50(12):1623–31.

[22] Davis K, Branson RD, Campbell RS, et al. Comparison of volume control and pressure control
ventilation: is flow waveform the difference?
J Trauma 1996;41:808–14.

[23] Laubscher TP, Frutiger A, Fanconi S, et al. Automatic selection of tidal volume, respiratory
frequency and minute volume in intubated ICU
patients as startup procedure for closed-loop
controlled ventilation. Int J Clin Monit Comput
1994;11:19–30.

[24] Laubscher TP, Frutiger A, Fanconi S, et al. The
automatic selection of ventilation parameters during
the initial phase of mechanical ventilation. Intensive
Care Med 1996;22:199–207.

[25] Campbell RS, Sinamban RP, Johannigman JA, et al.
Clinical evaluation of a new closed loop ventilation
mode: adaptive support ventilation. Respir Care
1998;43:856 [abstract].

[26] Arnal JM, Nafati C, Wysocki M, et al. Utilization of
an automatic mode of ventilation (ASV) in a mixed
ICU population: prospective observational study.
Intensive Care Med 2004;30:S84 [abstract].

[27] Tassaux D, Dalmas E, Gratadour P, et al. Patient-
ventilator interactions during partial ventilatory
support: a preliminary study comparing the effects
of adaptive support ventilation with synchronized
intermittent mandatory ventilation plus inspiratory
pressure support. Crit Care Med 2002;30:801–7.

[28] Sultzer CF, Chioléro R, Chassot PG, et al. Adaptive
support ventilation for tracheal extubation after cardiac surgery. Anesthesiology 2001;95:1339–45.

[29] Petter AH, Chiolero RL, Cassina T, et al. Automatic
"respirator/weaning" with adaptive support
ventilation: the effect on duration of endotracheal
intubation and patient management. Anesth Analg
2003;97:1743–50.

[30] Iotti GA, Belliato M, Polito A, et al. Safety and
effectiveness of adaptive support ventilation (ASV)
in acute respiratory failure. Intensive Care Med
2005;31:S168.

[31] Arnal JM, Wysocki M, Nafati C, et al. Automatic
selection of breathing pattern using adaptive
support ventilation. Intensive Care Med 2008;34:
75–81.

ELSEVIER
SAUNDERS

Clin Chest Med 29 (2008) 351–356

CLINICS
IN CHEST
MEDICINE

Index

Note: Page numbers of article titles are in **boldface** type.

A

Acute lung injury
  APRV in, **270–273.** See also *Airway pressure release ventilation (APRV), in acute lung injury and ARDS.*
  described, 233
  HFOV in, **265–275.** See also *High frequency oscillatory ventilation (HFOV), in acute lung injury and ARDS.*
  low tidal volume ventilation in, comparing and contrasting trials of, 225–226
  mechanical ventilatory support for, PEEP in, setting of, **233–239**
  mortality associated with, 265

Acute respiratory distress syndrome (ARDS)
  APRV in, **265–275.** See also *Airway pressure release ventilation (APRV), in acute lung injury and ARDS.*
  HFOV in, **265–275.** See also *High frequency oscillatory ventilation (HFOV), in acute lung injury and ARDS.*
  mortality associated with, 265

Acute Respiratory Distress Syndrome Network (ARDS-Net), 306, 307

Acute Respiratory Distress Syndrome (ARDS) Predictive Score, 260

Adapter devices, in aerosol medication delivery in mechanically ventilated patients, 280–282

Adaptive pressure control
  adaptive support vs., 346
  defined, 344

Adaptive support, adaptive pressure control vs., 346

Adaptive support ventilation, 344–345

Aerochamber HC, in aerosol medication delivery in mechanically ventilated patients, 281–282

Aerosol generator, in mechanically ventilated patients, 279–285

chlorofluorocarbon vs. hydrofluoroalkane pMDIs, 279–280
nebulizers, 282–284
pMDIs, 279–280
spacer or adapter devices, 280–282

Aerosol medications, for mechanically ventilated patients, delivery methods, **277–296**
  aerosol generator in, 279–285. See also *Aerosol generator, in mechanically ventilated patients.*
  aerosol particle size and, 285
  artificial airway and, 286–288
  device selection, 284–285
  during NPPV, 281
  efficiency of, 288–289
  factors influencing, 287–289
  gas density and, 285–286
  humidity and, 285
  inhalation therapy, clinical outcomes of, 289–290
  patient positioning for, 279
  synchronizing aerosol generation with inspiratory airflow, 288
  technique, 289
  ventilator breath characteristics, 288
  ventilator circuit conditions, 285–286
  ventilatory parameters, 288

Aerovent spacer, in aerosol medication delivery in mechanically ventilated patients, 281

Afferent(s), muscle, neural feedback from, in PAV and NAVA, 332

Airborne epidemic, mechanical ventilation in, **323–328.** See also *Mechanical ventilation, in airborne epidemic.*

Airway(s)
  artificial, in aerosol medication delivery for mechanically ventilated patients, 286–288
  upper, neural feedback from, in PAV and NAVA, 331–332

alveoli performance–related information from, 302

chest wall–related information from, 302

described, 300–302

inflation vs. deflation curves, 302–303

measurement of, 303–304

technical difficulties associated with, 303–304

ventilators in generation of, procedure, 304–305

Proportion assist ventilation (PAV), **329–342**
integration of mechanical ventilator in, 332–338
assist delivery in, 335–338
cycling-off assist in, 334–335
expiration in, 338
triggering of assist in, 332–334
neural feedback from respiratory system in, 331–332
transmission of respiratory motoneuron output to ventilation in, 330–331

Protocol(s), defined, 242

Protocol-driven ventilator weaning, **241–252**
concerns related to, 244–246
defined, 241–242
rationale supporting use of, 242–244
review of evidence for, 246–250
terminology related to, 242
"wake up and breathe" protocol, 249

Puritan Bennett 700 and 800 series, in aerosol medication delivery in mechanically ventilated patients, 284

R

Respiratory motoneuron output, transmission to ventilation, 330–331

Respiratory system, neural feedback from, in PAV and NAVA, 331–332

Respiratory-therapist driven protocols, on house-staff knowledge and education of mechanical ventilation, **313–321**. See also *Mechanical ventilation, house-sta knowledge and education of, respiratory-therapist driven protocols on.*

RTube, 308–309

S

SARS. See *Severe acute respiratory syndrome (SARS).*

Severe acute respiratory syndrome (SARS)
described, 323

in health care workers, protection techniques, 325

lessons from, 323–324

mechanical ventilation in, strategies for, 324–325

pandemic scenario and preparations, 325–326

prevalence of, 323

Society of Critical Care Medicine, 313

Spacer devices, in aerosol medication delivery in mechanically ventilated patients, 280–282

Stress index, pressure-time curves and, in mechanical ventilation, 305–306

SUN 345, in aerosol medication delivery in mechanically ventilated patients, 304

T

Tidal volume
for mechanical ventilatory support, setting of, **225–231**
operationalizing data in, 226–229
low, in acute lung injury, comparing and contrasting trials of, 225–226
selection of, overstretch injury concept in, 225

Tracheotomy, **253–263**
benefits of, 253–256
patient comfort, 253–254
secure airway, 254
VAP-related, 254–255
weaning from mechanical ventilation, 255
work of breathing, 255–256
complications related to, 256–257
contraindications to, 256
impact on outcome in critically ill patients, 257–258
indications for, 253
risks associated with, 256–257
techniques of, 256

U

Ultrasonic nebulizers, in aerosol medication delivery in mechanically ventilated patients, 283–284

Upper airways, neural feedback from, in PAV and NAVA, 331–332

V

VAP. See *Ventilator associated pneumonia (VAP).*

Ventilation